Upper Limb Movement Myotome and Peripheral Nerve Supply

Joint Movement	Muscle	Root	Peripheral Nerve
Shoulder abduction	Deltoid	C4/C5	Axillary
Shoulder adduction	Pectoralis/ latissimus dorsi	C6-C8	Medial and lateral pectoral
Elbow flexion	Biceps	C5/C6	Musculocutaneous
Elbow extension	Triceps	C7/C8	Radial
Wrist flexion	Flexor muscles of forearm	C7/C8	Median and ulnar
Wrist extension	Extensor muscles of forearm	C7	Radial
Digit flexion	Long finger flexors	C8	Median and ulnar
Digit extension	Long finger extensors	C7	Radial/posterior interosseous
Digit abduction	Intrinsic muscles of hand	T1	Median and ulnar

Lower Limb Movement Myotome and Peripheral Nerve Supply

Joint Movement	Muscle	Root	Peripheral Nerve
Hip abduction	Gluteal muscles	L4-S1	Sciatic
Hip adduction	Adductors	L2/L3	Obturator
Hip flexion	Iliopsoas (anterior compartment muscles)	L1-L3	Femoral
Hip extension	Gluteal and posterior compartment muscles	L5/S1	Sciatic
Knee flexion	Hamstrings	L5-S1	Sciatic
Knee extension	Quadriceps	L3/L4	Femoral
Ankle dorsiflexion	Anterior tibial	L4/L5	Common peroneal
Ankle plantar-flexion	Gastrocnemius and soleus	S1/S2	Tibial
Toe flexion	Flexor hallucis longus	S2/S3	Tibial
Toe extension	Extensor hallucis longus	L5/S1	Common peroneal

CHURCHILL'S POCKETBOOKS

Orthopaedics, Trauma and Rheumatology

Commissioning Editor: Alison Taylor
Development Editor: Janice Urquhart
Project Manager: Frances Affleck
Designer: Erik Bigland
Illustrations Manager: Merlyn Harvey
Illustrator: Amanda Williams

CHURCHILL'S POCKETBOOKS

Orthopaedics, Trauma and Rheumatology

Andrew D. Duckworth MB ChB BSc
Foundation Doctor, Accident and Emergency
Department, St John's Hospital, Livingston,
Scotland, UK

Daniel E. Porter MD FRCS (Orth)
Consultant Orthopaedic Surgeon, Royal Infirmary
of Edinburgh; Senior Lecturer, University of
Edinburgh, Edinburgh, Scotland, UK

Stuart H. Ralston MD FRCP FMedSci FRSE
Head of the School of Molecular and Clinical
Medicine and ARC Professor of Rheumatology,
Molecular Medicine Centre, Western General
Hospital, Edinburgh, Scotland UK

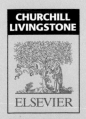

CHURCHILL
LIVINGSTONE

ELSEVIER

EDINBURGH LONDON NEW YORK OXFORD
PHILADELPHIA ST LOUIS SYDNEY TORONTO 2009

CHURCHILL
LIVINGSTONE
ELSEVIER

© 2009, Elsevier Limited. All rights reserved.

First published 2009
  Reprinted 2009

ISBN 9780443068492

British Library Cataloguing in Publication Data
A catalogue record for this book is available from the British Library

Library of Congress Cataloging in Publication Data
A catalog record for this book is available from the Library of Congress

Notice
Knowledge and best practice in this field are constantly changing. As new research and experience broaden our knowledge, changes in practice, treatment and drug therapy may become necessary or appropriate. Readers are advised to check the most current information provided (i) on procedures featured or (ii) by the manufacturer of each product to be administered, to verify the recommended dose or formula, the method and duration of administration, and contraindications. It is the responsibility of the practitioner, relying on their own experience and knowledge of the patient, to make diagnoses, to determine dosages and the best treatment for each individual patient, and to take all appropriate safety precautions. To the fullest extent of the law, neither the Publisher nor the authors assume any liability for any injury and/or damage to persons or property arising out of or related to any use of the material contained in this book.

The Publisher

PREFACE

There are many excellent undergraduate orthopaedic, rheumatology and trauma textbooks available to medical students. However, in the experience of the authors, there is no one publication that first of all covers all three topics suitable for the level of a trainee doctor, and secondly, is published in a format that fits in the lab coat pocket. This pocketbook aims to fulfil this role.

The text is aimed primarily at medical undergraduates for use during their placements in orthopaedics, A&E, rheumatology and general practice, as well as during their musculoskeletal anatomy course. The handbook is set up to provide the essential points for each region with regard to anatomy, examination, trauma and elective orthopaedics, whilst also providing information and succinct illustrations where suitable

The purpose of this text is not to replace the current recommended undergraduate texts within this speciality. It has the ambition of providing an affordable pocket size adjunct to these texts, whilst also imparting much of the core knowledge needed as an undergraduate.

A.D.D.
D.E.P.
S.H.R.

ACKNOWLEDGEMENTS

The authors would like to thank Dr Gordon Findlater and Dr Fanny Kristmundottir for their advice with the Anatomy section of the book. We are also indebted to Dr Simon Maxwell for his suggestions with the Therapeutics section of the book.

We would like to thank the Borders General Hospital Radiological Department and Dr Bethany Threlfall for their help with acquiring most of the radiographs seen throughout the text.

We are also indebted to Dr Mike Ford for allowing us to use the pictures from his text *An Introduction to Clinical Examination*.

Finally, we would like to thank Ann Duckworth, Nicola Duckworth, James Richards and Catherine Collinson for their hours of help in the preparation of this publication.

CONTENTS

ACRONYMS*

ABC airway, breathing, circulation

ACE angiotensin converting enzyme

ACL anterior cruciate ligament

ALP alkaline phosphatase

ANA antinuclear antibody

ANCA antineutrophil cytoplasmic antibody

AP anteroposterior

ARDS acute respiratory distress syndrome

ARF acute renal failure

AS ankylosing spondylitis

BMD bone mineral density

CCP cyclic citrullinated peptide

CK creatine kinase

CMCJ carpometacarpal joint

COX cyclo-oxygenase

CPDA common palmar digital artery

CRP c-reactive protein

CVA cerebrovascular accident

DDH developmental dysplasia of the hip

DEXA dual energy X-ray absorptiometry

DIC disseminated intravascular coagulation

DIPJ distal interphalangeal joint

DMARDs disease-modifying antirheumatic drugs

dsDNA double-stranded DNA

EPL extensor pollicis longus

FFD fixed flexion deformity

FOOSH fall onto the palmar aspect of the hand literally: fall onto outstretched hand

GCA giant cell arteritis

HBV hepatitis B virus

HRT hormone replacement therapy

IBD inflammatory bowel disease

IBS irritable bowel syndrome

Ig immunoglobulin

IHD ischaemic heart disease

IPJ interphalangeal joint

JIA juvenile idiopathic arthritis

LCL lateral collateral ligament

LFTs liver function tests

LMWH low molecular weight heparin

MCL medial collateral ligament

MCPJ metacarpophalangeal joint

MTPJ metatarsophalangeal joint

NICE National Institute for Health and Clinical Excellence

* All acronyms used in this book are listed here unless the acronym is well known (e.g. CNS, ECG, MRI), has been used only once, or has been used only in figures or tables, in which case the acronym is defined in the figure legend or at the end of the table.

NSAIDs non-steroidal anti-inflammatory drugs

OA osteoarthritis

ORIF open reduction and internal fixation

PA posteroanterior

PAN polyarteritis nodosa

PCL posterior cruciate ligament

PIPJ proximal interphalangeal joint

PMR polymyalgia rheumatica

PPI proton pump inhibitor

PsA psoriatic arthritis

PTH parathyroid hormone

RA rheumatoid arthritis

RF rheumatoid factor

ROM range of motion

RTA road traffic accident

SLE systemic lupus erythematosus

TNF tumour necrosis factor

USS ultrasound scan

VTE venous thromboembolism

WHO World Health Organization

ANATOMY

SHOULDER

BONES AND JOINTS (Figure 1.1)

The pectoral girdle has three joints:

- The sternoclavicular joint (atypical saddle-type synovial fibrocartilage joint):
  - is stabilized by the costoclavicular and sternoclavicular (anterior and posterior) ligaments
  - is innervated by the medial supraclavicular nerve
  - is supplied by the suprascapular and internal thoracic arteries.
- The acromioclavicular joint (atypical plane-type synovial fibrocartilage joint):

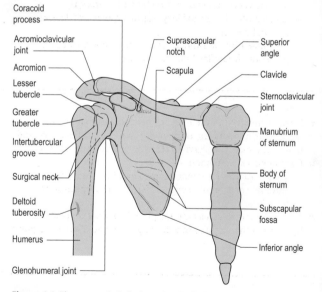

Figure 1.1 The pectoral girdle (anterior view). Fractures of the clavicle commonly occur two-thirds of the way along laterally. Fractures of the humerus commonly take place at the surgical neck. The **anatomical neck** is located between the humeral head and the tubercles. The bicipital groove separates the tubercles, and the **surgical neck** marks the border between the proximal humerus and the humeral shaft.

- is stabilized by the acromioclavicular and coracoclavicular ligaments
- is innervated by the lateral pectoral, supraclavicular and axillary nerves
- is supplied by the suprascapular and internal thoracic arteries.

● The shoulder (glenohumeral) joint:
- is a synovial ball and socket joint, with the head of the humerus articulating within the scapula's glenoid fossa:
  a. the shallow cavity is bordered by a lip of fibrocartilage known as the glenoid labrum that stabilizes the joint
  b. the joint is encompassed within a flexible capsule, which runs from the glenoid labrum around to the anatomical neck
  c. the capsule is reinforced by the rotator cuff tendons, the long head of biceps and the surrounding ligaments (glenohumeral, coracoacromial, coracohumeral, transverse humeral) but is still weak inferiorly
- is innervated by the axillary, suprascapular and lateral pectoral nerves
- is supplied by the suprascapular, and the anterior and posterior circumflex humeral arteries.

MUSCLES (Table 1.1 and Figure 1.2)

● Muscles involved in the movement of the scapula are levator scapulae, rhomboideus major and minor, pectoralis major and minor, trapezius, subclavius (clavicle) and serratus anterior
● Glenohumeral abduction:
- greater tuberosity impinges on glenoid labrum (~90°)
- external rotation of arm provides further abduction to 90–120°.
● Trapezius and serratus anterior provide abduction past ~120° by rotating the scapula, thus forcing the glenoid cavity to point superiorly.

BLOOD SUPPLY

The axillary artery supplies the shoulder region and:

● The origin is the subclavian artery, and it starts at the lateral border of the 1st rib surrounded by the axillary vein, lymph nodes and brachial plexus cords

TABLE 1.1 The muscles, with their innervations which provide movement at the shoulder joint*

Movement	Muscle	Origin	Insertion	Nerve
Abduction	Supraspinatus	Supraspinatus fossa of scapula	Greater tuberosity of humerus	Suprascapular
	Deltoid (m)	Acromion	Deltoid tuberosity of humerus	Axillary
Adduction	Latissimus dorsi	T6–T12, Iliac crest, Inferior ribs	Bicipital groove of humerus	Thoracodorsal
	Pectoralis major	Clavicle, sternum, upper six ribs	Bicipital groove of humerus	Pectoral nerves.
	Teres major	Posterior–inferior aspect of scapula	Medial lip of humeral bicipital groove	Subscapular
	Coracobrachialis	Coracoid process of scapula	Medial aspect of humeral shaft	Musculocutaneous
	Subscapularis	Subscapular fossa	Lesser tubercle of humerus	Subscapular
Flexion	Deltoid (a)	Lateral third of clavicle	Deltoid tuberosity of humerus	Axillary
	Pectoralis major	Clavicle, sternum, upper six ribs	Bicipital groove of humerus	Pectoral nerves.
	Coracobrachialis	Coracoid process of scapula	Medial aspect of humeral shaft	Musculocutaneous
Extension	Latissimus dorsi	T6–T12, Iliac crest, inferior ribs	Bicipital groove of humerus	Thoracodorsal
	Deltoid (p)	Spine of scapula	Deltoid tuberosity of humerus	Axillary
	Pectoralis major	Clavicle, sternum, upper six ribs	Bicipital groove of humerus	Pectoral nerves.
Medial rotation	Latissimus dorsi	T6–T12, iliac crest, inferior ribs	Bicipital groove of humerus	Thoracodorsal
	Pectoralis major	Clavicle, sternum, upper six ribs	Bicipital groove of humerus	Pectoral nerves.
	Teres major	Posterior–inferior aspect of scapula	Medial lip of humeral bicipital groove	Subscapular
	Deltoid (a)	Lateral third of clavicle	Deltoid tuberosity of humerus	Axillary
	Subscapularis	Subscapular fossa	Lesser tuberosity of humerus	Subscapular
Lateral rotation	Deltoid (p)	Spine of scapula	Deltoid tuberosity of humerus	Axillary
	Teres minor	Lateral border of scapula	Greater tuberosity of humerus	Axillary
	Infraspinatus	Infraspinous fossa of scapula	Greater tuberosity of humerus	Suprascapular

* Pectoralis major contributes to both shoulder flexion and extension, and is innervated by the lateral and medial pectoral nerves. It has two heads: clavicular (shoulder flexion) and sternocostal (shoulder extension). Coracobrachialis, an anterior compartment muscle of the arm, provides minor contributions to shoulder flexion and adduction.

a, anterior fibres of deltoid; m, middle fibres of deltoid; p, posterior fibres of deltoid.

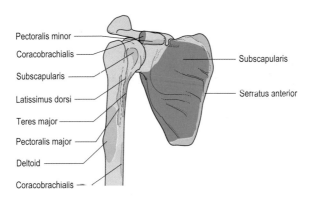

(Anterior aspect)

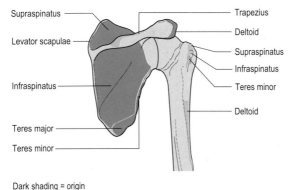

Dark shading = origin
Light shading = insertion

(Posterior aspect)

Figure 1.2 The muscles that contribute to movement at the shoulder joint.

- Branches include the superior thoracic artery, thoracoacromial artery, lateral thoracic artery, subscapular artery and circumflex humeral arteries (anterior and posterior)
- Becomes the brachial artery at the inferior edge of teres major.

BRACHIAL PLEXUS (Figure 1.3)

- The brachial plexus innervates the shoulder region as well as the rest of the upper limb.

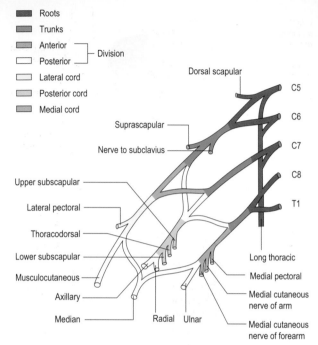

▮	Roots
▮	Trunks
▮	Anterior
▯	Posterior
▯	Lateral cord
▮	Posterior cord
▮	Medial cord

Division

Dorsal scapular

C5
C6
C7
C8
T1

Suprascapular

Nerve to subclavius

Upper subscapular

Lateral pectoral

Thoracodorsal

Lower subscapular

Long thoracic

Musculocutaneous

Medial pectoral

Axillary

Medial cutaneous nerve of arm

Median

Radial   Ulnar

Medial cutaneous nerve of forearm

Figure 1.3 The brachial plexus. (NB: Hilton's law states that the nerve that innervates a joint often innervates the overlying skin, as well as the muscles that move the joint.)

- The axillary nerve runs inferiorly to deltoid with the circumflex humeral arteries around the surgical neck of humerus and:
    — arises from the C5/6 roots and the posterior cord of the brachial plexus
    — gives sensory cutaneous divisions to the lateral aspect of the upper arm i.e. over deltoid
    — gives muscular innervations to deltoid and teres minor.

ARM AND ELBOW

BONES AND JOINTS (Figure 1.4)

The elbow joint:

- Is a hinged synovial joint that comprises three articular points:

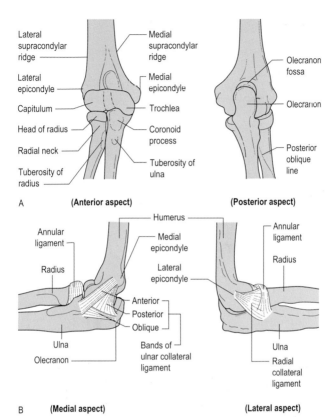

Figure 1.4 (A) Bones of the arm and elbow joint. Both epicondyles are extracapsular. (B) The elbow joint is stabilized by surrounding collateral and annular ligaments.

— medially, the humeral trochlea articulates with the ulnar's trochlear notch
— laterally, the proximal radial head articulates with the humeral capitulum
— and the proximal radioulnar joint (see p. 13).
- Is encompassed within a flexible capsule, which is weaker anteriorly and posteriorly but is reinforced by the radial (laterally) and ulnar (medially) collateral ligaments
- Is innervated by the radial and musculocutaneous nerves, with small contributions from the median and ulnar nerves.

MUSCLES (Table 1.2 and Figure 1.5)

The arm has an anterior and a posterior compartment divided by septa (medial and lateral intermuscular septa) formed from the deep fascia.

● Anterior (flexor) compartment (biceps brachii, brachialis, coracobrachialis):
— is innervated by the musculocutaneous nerve, apart from brachialis which is also supplied by the radial nerve

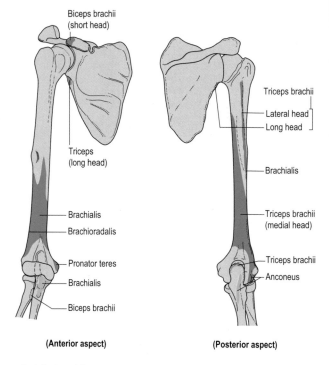

(Anterior aspect)   **(Posterior aspect)**

Dark shade = origin
Light shade = insertion

Figure 1.5 The muscles that contribute to movement at the elbow joint. The **antecubital fossa** is bordered by pronator teres (medially), brachioradialis (laterally) and brachialis and supinator (inferiorly/floors). It contains the brachial artery and the median nerve (medially). The radial nerve is sometimes considered part of the antecubital fossa.

TABLE 1.2 The muscles, with their innervations, which provide movement at the elbow joint*

Movement	Muscle	Origin	Insertion	Nerve
Elbow flexion	Biceps brachii			Musculocutaneous
	Long	Supraglenoid tuberosity	Radial tuberosity	
	Short	Coracoid process	Radial tuberosity	
	Brachialis	Anterior aspect of humerus	Ulnar coronoid process and tuberosity	Musculocutaneous, radial
	Pronator teres	Common flexor origin and coronoid process of ulnar	Lateral aspect of radius	Median
	Brachioradialis	Lateral supracondyle of humerus	Distal radius (styloid process)	Radial
Elbow extension	Triceps brachii			Radial
	Long	Infraglenoid tubercle of scapula	Olecranon process of ulna	
	Lateral, medial	Posterior aspect of humerus	Olecranon process of ulna	
	Anconeus	Lateral epicondyle of humerus	Olecranon process and shaft of ulna	Radial

* Pronation and supination of the forearm do not occur at the elbow (see Table 1.5). Brachioradialis (a posterior compartment muscle of the forearm) and the humeral head of pronator teres (an anterior compartment muscle of the forearm) both contribute to elbow flexion. Anconeus, a posterior compartment muscle of the forearm, contributes to elbow extension.

— biceps brachii has two heads (long and short) and is the strongest muscle responsible for forearm supination
— coracobrachialis contributes to shoulder flexion and adduction alone.
- Posterior (extensor) compartment (triceps):
  — is innervated by the radial nerve
  — triceps has three heads (long, medial and lateral).

BLOOD SUPPLY

The brachial artery supplies both the anterior and posterior compartments of the arm:

- The origin is the axillary artery and it starts at the inferior edge of teres major
- It branches to give:
  — profunda brachii that runs in the humeral spiral groove and supplies both compartments of the arm
  — superior and inferior ulnar collateral arteries that help supply the elbow joint.
- It becomes the radial and ulnar arteries at the radial neck (early/high bifurcation possible).

NERVES

- The musculocutaneous nerve (Figure 1.6) runs down the arm innervating the anterior compartment of the arm. It turns into the lateral cutaneous nerve of the forearm
- The radial nerve (Figure 1.7) runs in the humeral spiral groove with the profunda brachii vessels innervating the posterior compartment of the arm. It branches to give the posterior interosseous nerve, along with sensory cutaneous divisions to the posterior and lateral aspects of the arm, as well as the posterior forearm
- The median and ulnar nerves give off no branches in the arm. Of note, the ulnar nerve passes posterior to the humeral medial epicondyle in the ulnar groove (funny bone) of the elbow as it enters the forearm
- All four of these nerves (musculocutaneous, radial, median and ulnar) innervate the elbow joint and originate from the brachial plexus.

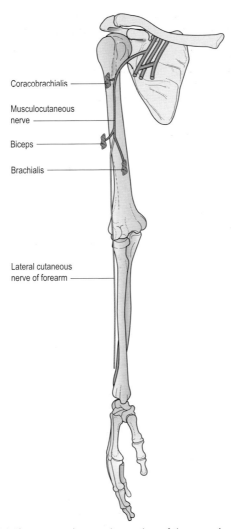

Figure 1.6 The motor and sensory innervations of the **musculocutaneous nerve**. It arises from the C5/6/7 roots and the lateral cord of the brachial plexus. It pierces coracobrachialis and then passes obliquely between biceps brachii and brachialis.

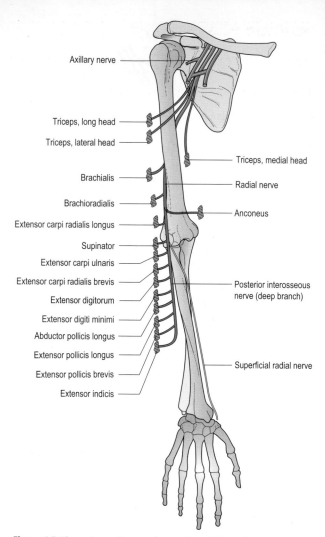

Figure 1.7 The motor and sensory innervations of the **radial nerve**. It arises from the C5/6/7/8 and T1 roots and the posterior cord of the brachial plexus. It then runs posterior to the axillary artery. It runs between the medial and long head of triceps, in the humeral spinal groove and then passes between brachialis and brachioradialis, running laterally to the biceps tendon and anterior to the lateral epicondyle.

FOREARM, WRIST AND HAND

BONES AND JOINTS (Figure 1.8)

The radioulnar joint is a pivot synovial joint and:

- Has a proximal and a distal joint, where pronation and supination occur
- Is innervated by:
  — proximal: median, radial and musculocutaneous nerves
  — distal: anterior and posterior interosseous nerves.
- Is supplied by the anterior and posterior interosseous arteries.

The wrist joint:

- Is a condyloid synovial joint and comprises:
  — the proximal carpal bones (triquetrum, lunate, scaphoid) with the distal radius and ulna, which are responsible predominantly for flexion/extension, abduction/adduction and circumduction of the wrist
  — the intercarpal joints are plane synovial joints, which are responsible predominantly for wrist abduction and flexion.
- Is reinforced by the ulnocarpal, radiocarpal and collateral ligaments
- Is innervated by the anterior interosseous (a branch of the median nerve) and the posterior interosseous (a branch of the radial nerve) nerves
- Is supplied by the palmar and dorsal carpal arterial arches.

The hand joints:

- Include the carpometacarpal joints (CMCJs), MCPJs, PIPJs and DIPJs
- Are all synovial joints.

MUSCLES (Figure 1.9)

The forearm has an anterior and a posterior compartment divided by a robust interosseous membrane that connects the radius and ulna.

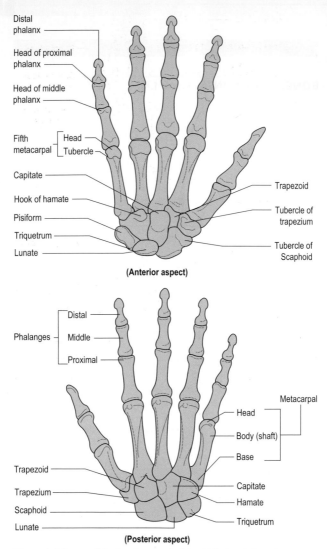

Figure 1.8 Bones of the hand and wrist joint (right hand shown).

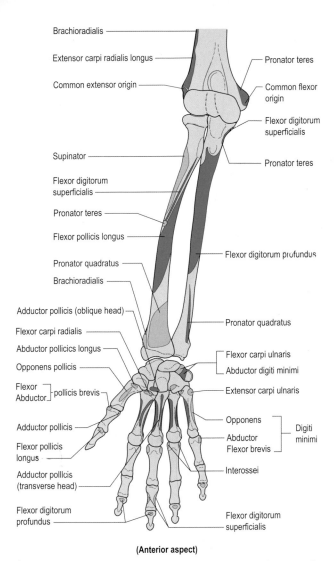

(Anterior aspect)

Figure 1.9 The muscles that contribute to movement of the forearm and at the wrist and hand. The **common flexor origin** is found on the medial epicondyle of the humerus. The **common extensor origin** is found on the lateral epicondyle of the humerus. The long flexor tendons originate from muscles of the anterior compartment of the forearm and travel under the flexor retinaculum to insertion points on the metacarpal and phalanx bones via synovial flexor tendon sheaths.

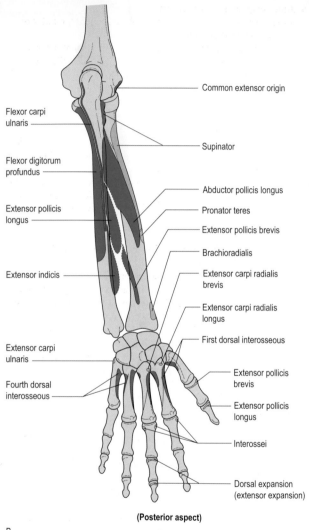

Common extensor origin

Flexor carpi ulnaris

Supinator

Flexor digitorum profundus

Abductor pollicis longus

Extensor pollicis longus

Pronator teres

Extensor pollicis brevis

Brachioradialis

Extensor indicis

Extensor carpi radialis brevis

Extensor carpi radialis longus

First dorsal interosseous

Extensor carpi ulnaris

Extensor pollicis brevis

Fourth dorsal interosseous

Extensor pollicis longus

Interossei

Dorsal expansion (extensor expansion)

(Posterior aspect)

B

Figure 1.9, cont'd The long extensor tendons follow a similar path on the dorsal surface, again within synovial sheaths, and insert into the middle and distal phalanges. The palmar aponeurosis (anterior aspect) is a thick sheet that connects the thenar and hypothenar muscles across the hand; thickening and contracture of this leads to the characteristic deformity seen in Dupuytren's contracture.

- Anterior (flexor) compartment:
  — is innervated by the median (plus its branch, the anterior interosseous) and ulnar nerves
  — flexor carpi ulnaris (ulnar and humeral), pronator teres (ulnar and humeral) and flexor digitorum superficialis (radial and humeroulnar) all have two heads
  — is predominantly responsible for flexion of the wrist (Table 1.3), as well as flexion of the digital joints (Table 1.4)
  — flexor digitorum superficialis and flexor digitorum profundus are responsible for digital flexion (excluding the thumb) via attachment of long flexor tendons to the middle phalanx and terminal phalanx, respectively
  — is also responsible for pronation of the forearm (Table 1.5) with pronator quadratus contributing to forearm pronation alone, whereas pronator teres also contributes to elbow flexion.
- Posterior (extensor) compartment:
  — is innervated by the radial nerve and its branch, the posterior interosseous nerve
  — is predominantly responsible for extension of the wrist joint (Table 1.3), as well as extension of the digital joints; it also contributes to thumb extension and abduction (Table 1.4)
  — is also responsible for supination of the forearm (Table 1.5) with supinator aiding biceps brachii
  — brachioradialis contributes to elbow flexion alone, whereas anconeus contributes to elbow extension alone.

The intrinsic muscles of the hand are often explained using three definable groups:

- Thenar eminence (abductor pollicis brevis, flexor pollicis brevis, opponens pollicis):
  — is innervated by the recurrent branch of the median nerve
  — is responsible for movements of the thumb (Table 1.4)
- Hypothenar eminence (abductor digiti minimi, flexor digiti minimi, opponens digiti minimi):
  — is innervated by the deep branch of the ulnar nerve
  — is responsible for movements of the little finger (Table 1.4).
- Other intrinsic muscles (palmar interossei, dorsal interossei, lumbricals, adductor pollicis):

TABLE 1.3 The muscles, with their innervations, which provide movement at the wrist joint*

Movement	Muscle	Origin	Insertion	Nerve
Wrist abduction	Extensor carpi radialis longus (PS)	Lateral supracondyle of humerus	2nd metacarpal base	Radial
	Extensor carpi radialis brevis (PS)	Common extensor origin	3rd metacarpal base	Posterior interosseous
	Flexor carpi radialis (AS)	Common flexor origin	2nd metacarpal base	Median
Wrist adduction	Flexor carpi ulnaris (AS) Humeral head Ulnar head	Common flexor origin Olecranon and posterior ulnar	Pisiform/5th metacarpal Pisiform/5th metacarpal	Ulnar
	Extensor carpi ulnaris (PS)	Common extensor origin	5th metacarpal base	Posterior interosseous
Wrist flexion	Flexor carpi ulnaris (AS)	See above	See above	Ulnar
	Flexor carpi radialis (AS)	Common flexor origin	2nd metacarpal base	Median
	Palmaris longus (AS)	Common flexor origin	Palmar aponeurosis	Median
	Flexor digitorum superficialis (AS)	Common flexor origin, coronoid process, radius	4 ulnar middle phalanges	Median
	Flexor digitorum profundus (AD)	Ulnar and interosseous membrane	4 ulnar distal phalanges	Ulnar/anterior interosseous
Wrist extension	Extensor carpi radialis longus (PS)	Lateral supracondyle of humerus	2nd metacarpal base	Radial
	Extensor carpi radialis brevis (PS)	Common extensor origin	3rd metacarpal base	Posterior interosseous
	Extensor carpi ulnaris (PS)	Common extensor origin	5th metacarpal base	Posterior interosseous
	Extensor digitorum (PS)	Common extensor origin	Extensor expansions of 4 ulnar middle/distal phalanges	Posterior interosseous

* Flexor digitorum profundus is supplied by the ulnar nerve medially and the anterior interosseous nerve laterally.
A, anterior compartment of forearm; D, deep; P, posterior compartment of forearm; S, superficial.

TABLE 1.4 The muscles, with their innervations, which provide movement of the digital joints*

Movement	Muscle	Origin	Insertion	Nerve
Thumb abduction	Abductor pollicis longus (PD) Abductor pollicis brevis (TS)	Ulnar and radius Scaphoid, trapezium, FR	1st MC base Thumb proximal phalanx	Posterior interosseous Recurrent branch median
Thumb adduction	Adductor pollicis (I)	Capitate, trapezoid, 2nd/3rd MC	Thumb proximal phalanx	Deep branch ulnar
Thumb flexion	Flexor pollicis longus (AD) Flexor pollicis brevis (TS)	Radius and interosseous membrane Trapezium, FR	Thumb distal phalanx Thumb proximal phalanx	Anterior interosseous Recurrent branch median
Thumb extension	Extensor pollicis brevis (PD) Extensor pollicis longus (PD)	Radius and interosseous membrane Ulnar and interosseous membrane	Thumb proximal phalanx Thumb distal phalanx	Posterior interosseous Posterior interosseous
5th digit abduction	Abductor digiti minimi (HS)	Pisiform, FR	5th digit proximal phalanx	Deep branch ulnar
5th digit flexion	Flexor digiti minimi (HS)	Hook of hamate, FR	5th digit proximal phalanx	Deep branch ulnar
5th digit extension	Extensor digiti minimi (PS)	Common extensor origin	Extensor expansion of 5th digit	Posterior interosseous
Digital abduction	Dorsal interossei (I)	Metacarpals	Base proximal phalanges	Deep branch ulnar
Digital adduction	Palmar interossei (I)	Metacarpals	Base proximal phalanges	Deep branch ulnar
Digital flexion	FDS (AS) FDP (AD)	See Table 1.3 See Table 1.3	See Table 1.3 See Table 1.3	Median Ulnar/ anterior interosseous
Digital extension	Extensor digitorum (PS)	Common extensor origin	Extensor expansion 4 ulnar middle/distal phalanges	Posterior interosseous

*Extensor indicis, a posterior compartment muscle of the forearm, contributes to 2nd digit extension alone. Opponens pollicis and opponens digiti minimi medially rotate the thumb and 5th digit, respectively, creating opposition, thus producing a grip that is also aided by palmaris brevis. A, anterior compartment of forearm; D, deep; FDP, flexor digitorum profundus; FDS, flexor digitorum superficialis; FR, flexor retinaculum; H, hypothenar eminence; I, intrinsic muscle of hand; MC, metacarpal; P, posterior compartment of forearm; S, superficial; T, thenar eminence.

TABLE 1.5 The muscles, with their innervations, which provide movement at the radioulnar joint*

Movement	Muscle	Origin	Insertion	Nerve
Pronation	Pronator teres (AS) Humeral head Ulnar head	Common flexor origin Coronoid process of ulna	Lateral aspect of radius Lateral aspect of radius	Median
	Pronator quadratus (AD)	Anteromedial aspect of ulna	Anterolateral aspect of radius	Anterior interosseous
Supination	Supinator (PS)	Common extensor origin, elbow ligaments, crest of ulna	Radial neck and shaft	Posterior interosseous
	Biceps brachii	See Table 1.2	See Table 1.2	See Table 1.2

* Biceps brachii, an anterior compartment muscle of the arm, contributes to supination. Anconeus, a posterior compartment muscle of the forearm, contributes to movement of the ulna during pronation.

A, anterior compartment of forearm; D deep; P, posterior compartment of forearm; S, superficial.

— are innervated by the deep branch of the ulnar nerve and
the median nerve
— are responsible for abduction and adduction of the digits, as
well as MCPJ flexion/IPJ extension (Table 1.4). The
lumbricals do the latter also
— adductor pollicis is responsible for thumb adduction alone.

BLOOD SUPPLY (Figure 1.10)

The radial and ulnar arteries supply both the anterior and
posterior compartments of the forearm and the hand.

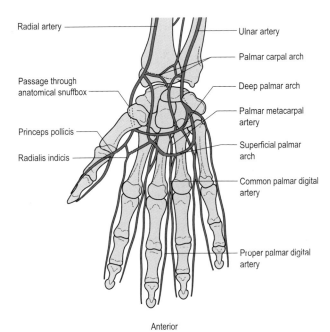

Anterior

Figure 1.10 The blood supply of the wrist joint and hand. The radial artery
runs between flexor carpi radialis and brachioradialis in the forearm. At the
wrist it is palpable. The ulnar artery runs inferior to the common flexor origin
and then between FDP and flexor carpi ulnaris in the forearm. It runs lateral
to the ulnar nerve in the distal forearm and wrist.

- The ulnar artery:
  — gives rise early to the common interosseous artery, which divides to produce the anterior interosseous artery and the posterior interosseous artery; these two vessels rejoin to supply the dorsum of the hand
  — enters the hand superficial to the flexor retinaculum to give rise to the superficial palmar arch, from where it supplies the digits via the CPDAs.
- The radial artery:
  — enters the hand via the anatomical snuffbox (deep to APL and EPB tendons) to give rise to the deep palmar arch, from where it supplies the digits via branches that anastomose with the CPDAs.

NERVES

- The median nerve (Figure 1.11) enters the forearm between the heads of pronator teres, innervating some of the muscles in the anterior compartment of the forearm. The nerve is superficial at the wrist and in the midline. It then enters the hand via the carpal tunnel (inferior to the flexor retinaculum and superolaterally to the tendons of FDS/FDP) and innervates the muscles of the thenar eminence as well as the 1st and 2nd (radial) lumbricals. Significant branches throughout this course include:
  — the anterior interosseous nerve, which innervates some of the muscles in the anterior compartment of the forearm
  — sensory cutaneous divisions to the central and radial aspect of the palm, and the radial 3½ digits (Figure 1.12).
- The ulnar nerve (Figure 1.13) enters the forearm between the heads of flexor carpi ulnaris, innervating some of the muscles in the anterior compartment of the forearm. It then enters the hand superficial to the flexor retinaculum and divides (deep and superficial) to innervate the remaining intrinsic muscles of the hand. Sensory cutaneous divisions innervate the medial palm and ulnar 1½ digits (Figure 1.12)
- The radial nerve (Figure 1.7) enters the forearm inferior to brachioradialis, innervating some of the muscles in the posterior compartment of the forearm. Significant branches throughout this course include:
  — the posterior interosseous nerve at the elbow (lateral epicondyle), which passes between the two heads of supinator and innervates some of the muscles in the posterior compartment of the forearm, as well as the wrist joint

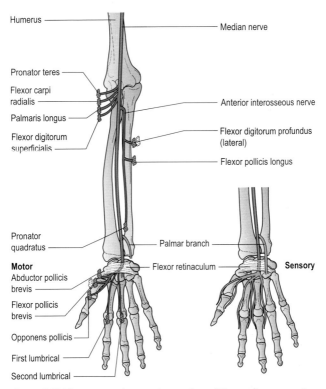

Humerus

Median nerve

Pronator teres

Flexor carpi radialis

Palmaris longus

Anterior interosseous nerve

Flexor digitorum superficialis

Flexor digitorum profundus (lateral)

Flexor pollicis longus

Pronator quadratus

Palmar branch

Motor

Flexor retinaculum

Sensory

Abductor pollicis brevis

Flexor pollicis brevis

Opponens pollicis

First lumbrical

Second lumbrical

Figure 1.11 The motor and sensory innervations of the **median nerve**. It arises from the C6/7/8 and T1 roots and the lateral and medial cords of the brachial plexus. Of note, the **median nerve** crosses the brachial artery in the arm (humeral shaft), moving from lateral to medial, both of which lie medial and superficial to the biceps tendon and brachialis respectively. After entering between the heads of pronator teres, in the forearm it runs between FDS and FDP and gives off the anterior interosseous nerve. It gives off the palmar branch (supplies skin over thenar eminence), which passes superior to the flexor retinaculum, just before the wrist.

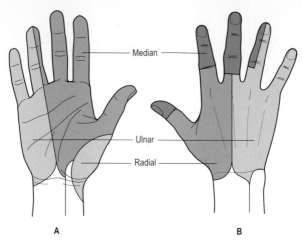

Figure 1.12 Sensory innervation of the hand: (A) anterior; (B) posterior.

— sensory cutaneous divisions to the lateral dorsum of the hand (Figure 1.12).

HIP, THIGH AND KNEE

BONES AND JOINTS

The hip joint (Figure 1.14):

● Is a highly stable synovial ball and socket joint that is covered with hyaline cartilage and comprises the femoral head articulating within the acetabulum of the pelvis, which is bordered by a lip of fibrocartilage known as the acetabular labrum that stabilizes the joint. Ligamention terres passes from the femoral head fovea to the margins of the acetabular notch
● Is encompassed within a flexible capsule, which is reinforced and stabilized by the surrounding ligaments (iliofemoral, puberofemoral, ischiofemoral)
● Is innervated by the sciatic, femoral and obturator nerves
● Is supplied by the obturator, medial and lateral circumflex femoral and the superior and inferior gluteal arteries (the latter four forming the trochanteric anastomosis).

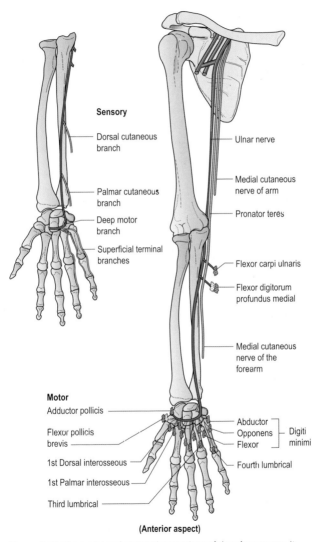

Sensory

Dorsal cutaneous branch

Palmar cutaneous branch

Deep motor branch

Superficial terminal branches

Ulnar nerve

Medial cutaneous nerve of arm

Pronator teres

Flexor carpi ulnaris

Flexor digitorum profundus medial

Medial cutaneous nerve of the forearm

Motor

Adductor pollicis

Flexor pollicis brevis

1st Dorsal interosseous

1st Palmar interosseous

Third lumbrical

Abductor ⎫
Opponens ⎬ Digiti
Flexor ⎭ minimi

Fourth lumbrical

(Anterior aspect)

Figure 1.13 The motor and sensory innervations of the **ulnar nerve**. It arises from the C7/8 and T1 roots and the medial cord of the plexus. The **ulnar nerve** runs anteromedially to the humerus between the axillary artery and vein, and then medially to the brachial artery, running anterior to the triceps. In the forearm it runs between FDP and flexor carpi ulnaris and medial to the ulnar artery.

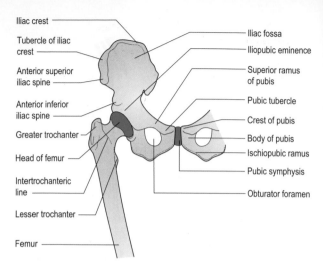

Figure 1.14 The hip joint is a stable and highly mobile ball and socket synovial joint. The sacrotuberous and sacrospinous ligaments form the greater and lesser sciatic foramens.

The knee joint (Figure 1.15):

- Is a synovial hinge joint that is covered with hyaline cartilage and comprises:
  - the femoral condyles articulating with the proximal tibial condyles
  - the patella articulating with femur.
- Is encompassed within a flexible incomplete capsule, which is reinforced and stabilized by tendons (e.g. from the quadriceps muscles), the surrounding ligaments (patella, LCL, MCL, ACL, PCL, oblique and arcuate popliteal), as well as the patella itself
- Has menisci, which are crescent-shaped mobile wedges that aid load bearing. They are found attached to the superior surface of the tibia and surrounding ligaments. Damage to the ligaments can lead to an associated meniscal tear
- Is innervated by the femoral, sciatic (tibial, common peroneal) and obturator nerves
- Is supplied by the branches from the genicular anastomoses (e.g. from the popliteal artery).

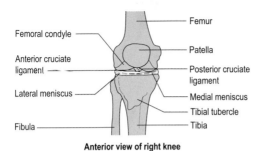

Anterior cruciate ligament
Femoral condyle
Femur
Patella
Posterior cruciate ligament
Lateral meniscus
Medial meniscus
Tibial tubercle
Fibula
Tibia

Anterior view of right knee

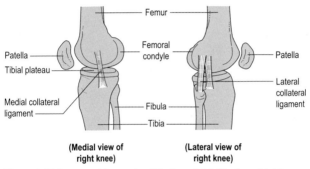

Femur
Femoral condyle
Patella
Tibial plateau
Patella
Lateral collateral ligament
Medial collateral ligament
Fibula
Tibia

(Medial view of right knee)   **(Lateral view of right knee)**

Figure 1.15 Bones and ligaments of the knee joint. The knee joint is surrounded by bursa. Of note is the suprapatellar bursa that has a direct link to the articular cavity; hence, inflammation of the knee joint can easily spread to this bursa. The gastrocnemius, anserine and popliteus bursae also communicate with the synovial cavity. The weaker ACL arises from the anterior intercondylar area of the tibia, runs obliquely and inserts into the posteromedial aspect of the lateral femoral condyle. PCL arises from the posterior intercondylar area of the tibia and inserts into the anterolateral aspect of the medial femoral condyle. The medial menisci is larger than the lateral.

MUSCLES (Figure 1.16)

The gluteal muscles are innervated by the superior or the inferior gluteal nerve, or the sacral plexus. Their prominent role is in hip abduction, along with medial and lateral rotation. The anterior fibres of gluteus medius provide a minor contribution to external rotation of the hip, whilst the posterior fibres provide a minor contribution to lateral rotation. Gluteus maximus contributes to hip extension.

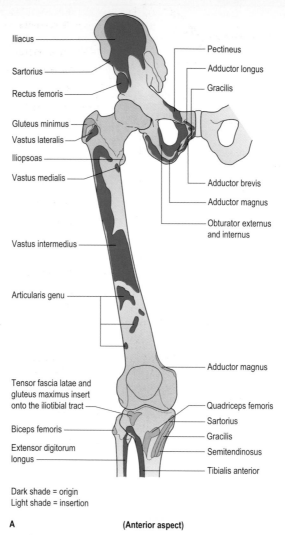

Iliacus

Sartorius

Rectus femoris

Gluteus minimus

Vastus lateralis

Iliopsoas

Vastus medialis

Vastus intermedius

Articularis genu

Tensor fascia latae and
gluteus maximus insert
onto the iliotibial tract

Biceps femoris

Extensor digitorum
longus

Pectineus

Adductor longus

Gracilis

Adductor brevis

Adductor magnus

Obturator externus
and internus

Adductor magnus

Quadriceps femoris

Sartorius

Gracilis

Semitendinosus

Tibialis anterior

Dark shade = origin
Light shade = insertion

A   (Anterior aspect)

Figure 1.16 The muscles that contribute to movement of the lower limb.
The **femoral triangle** contains the femoral nerve, artery, vein and canal (the
latter three encompassed within the femoral sheath), as well as the deep
inguinal lymph nodes. The borders of the triangle are the inguinal
ligament (superiorly), the adductor longus muscle (medially) and the
sartorius muscle (laterally). The borders of the **femoral ring** (entry point to
femoral canal) are the inguinal ligament (anteriorly), the lacunar ligament
(medially),

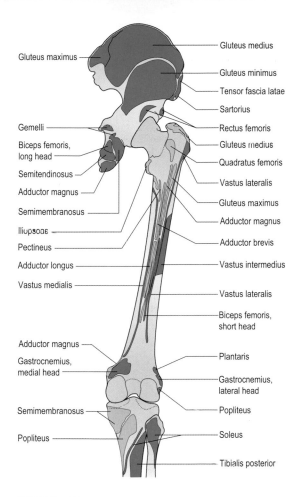

Dark shade = origin
Light shade = insertion

B (Posterior aspect)

Figure 1.16, cont'd the pectineal ligament (posteriorly) and the femoral vein (laterally). The **adductor canal** contains the femoral artery and vein, along with the saphenous nerve. The borders are sartorius (anteriomedially), vastus medialis (anterolaterally) and adductor longus and magnus (posteriorly/floor). The **popliteal fossa** involves the posterior aspect of the knee and contains the popliteal vessels, branches of the sciatic nerve, as well as lymph nodes and bursa. The borders of the fossa are semimembranous and semitendinosus (superomedially), biceps femoris (superolaterally), with the lateral and medial heads of gastrocnemius (inferiorly).

The thigh has three compartments – anterior, adductor and posterior – divided and encompassed by intermuscular septa and fascia lata, respectively.

- Anterior compartment (quadriceps femoris, psoas major, sartorius, iliacus, pectineus):
  — is innervated by the femoral nerve, apart from psoas major that is innervated by the lumbar plexus, and pectineus that is partially innervated by the obturator nerve
  — is responsible for movements at the hip and knee joint (Tables 1.6 and 1.7).
- Medial (adductor) compartment (adductor longus, brevis and magnus, obturator externus, gracilis):
  — is innervated by the obturator nerve, apart from adductor magnus that is also innervated by the sciatic nerve (tibial division)
  — is predominantly responsible for hip adduction (Tables 1.6 and 1.7)
  — the horizontal fibres of adductor magnus provide a minor contribution to hip flexion, whilst the vertical fibres provide a minor contribution to hip extension
  — adductor longus and brevis provide minor contributions to hip flexion.
- Posterior compartment (biceps femoris, semimembranosus, semitendinosus):
  — is innervated by the common peroneal and tibial divisions of the sciatic nerve
  — is responsible for hip extension, as well as knee flexion and rotation (Tables 1.6 and 1.7)
  — biceps femoris has two heads (long and short), with the long providing a minor contribution to hip extension.

BLOOD SUPPLY

- The superior (lies above piriformis as passes through foramen) and inferior gluteal arteries originate from the internal iliac artery and supply the gluteal muscles, as well as the hip joint. The internal pudendal artery also supplies some muscles of the gluteal region. All pass through the greater sciatic foramen
- The obturator artery originates from the internal iliac artery and supplies predominantly the adductor compartment of the thigh, as well as the hip joint

TABLE 1.6 The muscles, with their innervations, which provide movement at the hip joint

Movement	Muscle	Origin	Insertion	Nerve
Abduction	Gluteus medius (G)	Ilium	Greater trochanter of femur	Superior gluteal
	Gluteus minimus (G)	Ilium	Greater trochanter of femur	Superior gluteal
	Sup. and inf. gemellus (G)	Ischial spine and tuberosity	Greater trochanter of femur	L5/S1 (sacral plexus)
Adduction	Pectineus (A)	Superior pubic ramus	Lesser trochanter of femur	Femoral
	Adductor brevis (M)	Inferior pubic ramus	Posterior aspect of femur	Obturator
	Adductor longus (M)	Body of pubis	Posterior aspect of femur	Obturator
	Adductor magnus (M)	Ischiopubic ramus	Posterior aspect of femur	Obturator, sciatic
	Gracilis (M)	Ischiopubic ramus	Superior/medial aspect of tibia	Obturator
Medial rotation	Gluteus minimus (G)	Ilium	Greater trochanter of femur	Superior gluteal
	Tensor fascia lata (G)	Iliac crest and ASIS	Iliotibial tract	Superior gluteal
Lateral rotation	Quadratus femoris (G)	Ischial tuberosity	Intertrochanteric crest of femur	L5/S1 (sacral plexus)
	Obturator internus (G)	Obturator membrane	Greater trochanter of femur	L5/S1 (sacral plexus)
	Piriformis (G)	Anterior aspect of sacrum	Greater trochanter of femur	Piriformis
	Sartorius (A)	Anterior superior iliac spine	Superior/medial aspect of tibia	Femoral
	Obturator externus (M)	Obturator membrane	Greater trochanter of femur	Obturator
	Sup. and inf. gemellus (G)	Ischial spine and tuberosity	Greater trochanter of femur	L5/S1 (sacral plexus)
Flexion	Sartorius (A)	Anterior superior iliac spine	Tibia	Femoral
	Psoas major (A)	Spine (T12–L5)	Lesser trochanter of femur	L1–L3 (lumbar plexus)
	Iliacus (A)	Iliac crest and fossa	Lesser trochanter of femur	Femoral
	Pectineus (A)	Superior pubic ramus	Femoral shaft	Femoral
Extension	Gluteus maximus (G)	Ilium, coccyx, sacrum, sacrotuberous ligament	Gluteal tuberosity of the femur, iliotibial tract	Inferior gluteal
	Biceps femoris (P)	Ischial tuberosity and posterior aspect of femur	Fibula head	Tibial, common peroneal
	Semimembranosus (P)	Ischial tuberosity	Tibia (medial condyle)	Tibial
	Semitendinosus (P)	Ischial tuberosity	Tibia (superomedial aspect)	Tibial

A, anterior compartment of thigh; G, gluteal region; M, medial compartment of thigh. Those muscles attaching to the posterior aspect of the femur will predominantly do so via the linea aspera of the femur.

TABLE 1.7 The muscles, with their innervations, which provide movement at the knee joint*

Movement	Muscle	Origin	Insertion	Nerve
Flexion	Sartorius (A)	Anterior superior iliac spine	Superior/medial aspect of tibia	Femoral
	Gracilis (M)	Ischiopubic ramus	Superior/medial aspect of tibia	Obturator
	Biceps femoris (P)	Ischial tuberosity and posterior aspect of femur	Fibula head	Tibial, common peroneal
	Semimembranosus (P)	Ischial tuberosity	Tibia (medial condyle)	Tibial
	Semitendinosus (P)	Ischial tuberosity	Tibia (superomedial aspect)	Tibial
Extension	Rectus femoris (A)	Anterior inferior iliac spine	Patellar tendon onto tibia	Femoral
	Vastus medialis (A)	Upper aspect of femur	Patellar tendon onto tibia	Femoral
	Vastus lateralis (A)	Upper aspect of femur	Patellar tendon onto tibia	Femoral
	Vastus intermedius (A)	Body of femur	Patellar tendon onto tibia	Femoral

* The quadriceps is a group of muscles including vastus medialis, vastus lateralis, vastus intermedius and rectus femoris. Gastrocnemius and plantaris, posterior compartment muscles of the leg, provide minor contributions to knee flexion. The posterior compartment muscles are responsible for lateral and medial rotation of the knee joint when it is in flexion. Locking and unlocking of the knee are controlled by the surrounding ligaments and the popliteus muscle, respectively. A, anterior compartment of thigh; M, medial compartment of thigh; P, posterior compartment of thigh.

- The femoral artery supplies the anterior compartment of the thigh:
  — the origin is the external iliac artery and it starts at the inferior edge of the inguinal ligament
  — it gives rise to profunda femoris (susceptable in femoral shaft fractures) that supplies the posterior compartment of the thigh, and itself gives rise to the four perforating and the medial and lateral circumflex femoral arteries
  — it becomes the popliteal artery at the adductor magnus hiatus.
- The cruciate anastomosis (first perforator of deep femoral, inferior gluteal artery, medial and lateral circumflex femoral arteries) supply the posterior aspect of the femur and is a collateral blood supply if the femoral artery becomes compromised
- The popliteal artery:
  — gives rise to the superior, middle and inferior genicular artery branches, which supply the knee joint; it also gives rise to the sural arteries that supply some muscles of the leg
  — is susceptible to damage with a distal femoral fracture due to its bordering course
  — is the deepest structure of the popliteal fossa
  — becomes the anterior and posterior tibial arteries at the inferior edge of the popliteus muscle.

NERVES (Figure 1.17)

- The lumbar and sacral plexus innervates the lower limb
- The sacral plexus with the superior and inferior gluteal nerves, which pass through the greater sciatic foramen, predominantly innervate the gluteal muscles
- The femoral nerve (L2–L4) enters deep to the inguinal ligament innervating the anterior compartment of the thigh. Its branches include the saphenous nerve and sensory cutaneous divisions to the anterior and medial aspects of the thigh
- The obturator nerve (L2–L4) enters through the obturator foramen innervating the adductor compartment of the thigh, with sensory cutaneous divisions of the medial aspect of the thigh
- The sciatic nerve (L4–L5, S1–S3) enters through the greater sciatic foramen (inferior to piriformis) emerging deep to gluteus maximus it innervates the posterior compartment of the thigh with two divisions that occur just superior to the knee joint, the **common peroneal** and **tibial nerve**.

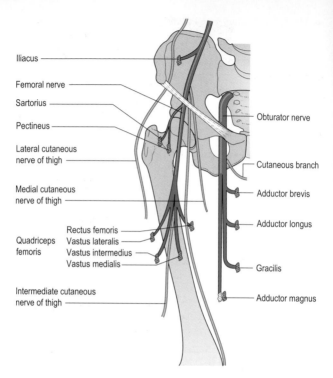

Iliacus

Femoral nerve

Sartorius

Pectineus

Lateral cutaneous nerve of thigh

Medial cutaneous nerve of thigh

Quadriceps femoris
- Rectus femoris
- Vastus lateralis
- Vastus intermedius
- Vastus medialis

Intermediate cutaneous nerve of thigh

Obturator nerve

Cutaneous branch

Adductor brevis

Adductor longus

Gracilis

Adductor magnus

A   **(Anterior aspect)**

Figure 1.17 The motor and sensory innervations of the hip and knee region. The greater and lesser sciatic foramen are formed through the sacrospinous and sacrotuberous ligaments transecting the sciatic notches. In the greater sciatic foramen, the superior gluteal vessels and nerve pass superior to piriformis. Branches of the **lumbar plexus** (L1–L4) include the femoral, obturator, genitofemoral and ilioinguinal nerves, along with the lateral cutaneous nerve of the thigh.

LEG AND FOOT

BONES AND JOINTS

The tibiofibular joint:

- Has proximal (superior) and distal (inferior) joints. The inferior joint is stabilized by the surrounding ligaments (anterior tibiofibular and posterior tibiofibular)

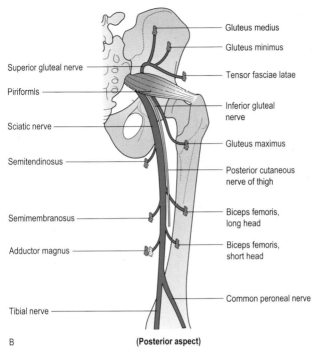

Gluteus medius

Gluteus minimus

Superior gluteal nerve

Tensor fasciae latae

Piriformis

Inferior gluteal nerve

Sciatic nerve

Gluteus maximus

Semitendinosus

Posterior cutaneous nerve of thigh

Semimembranosus

Biceps femoris, long head

Adductor magnus

Biceps femoris, short head

Common peroneal nerve

Tibial nerve

B   **(Posterior aspect)**

Figure 1.17, cont'd Branches of the **sacral plexus** (L4–L5, S1–S4) include the superior and inferior gluteal, sciatic pudendal and nerves, along with the posterior cutaneous nerve of the thigh.

- Is innervated by:
    - proximal: common peroneal nerve
    - distal: deep peroneal, saphenous and tibial nerves.
- Is supplied by:
    - proximal: anterior tibial and inferior lateral genicular arteries
    - distal: anterior and posterior tibial arteries.

The ankle joint (Figure 1.18):

- Is a stable hinged synovial joint covered with cartilage and comprises:
    - the distal inferior surfaces of the fibula and tibia (the lateral and medial malleoli, respectively) articulating with the superior surface body of the talus bone.

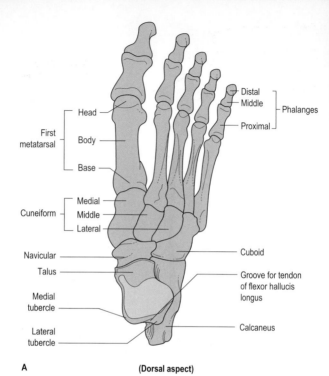

Figure 1.18 (A) Anatomy of the foot. The longitudinal (medial and lateral) and transverse arches of the foot aid in weight bearing and walking. The medial longitudinal arch includes the calcaneus, talus, navicular, three cuneiforms and the three medial metatarsals. The lateral longitudinal arch includes the calcaneus, cuboid and two lateral metatarsals. The transverse arch includes the proximal metatarsals as well as the three cuneiforms and the cuboid.

- Is encompassed within a loose capsule, which is reinforced and stabilized by the surrounding ligaments in order of strength:
  — medial or deltoid ligament
  — lateral ligaments (anterior and posterior talofibular, calcaneofibular).
- Is more stable in dorsiflexion due to the wider anterior–superior surface of the talus bone
- Is innervated by the deep peroneal and tibial nerves
- Is supplied by the anterior and posterior tibial arteries.

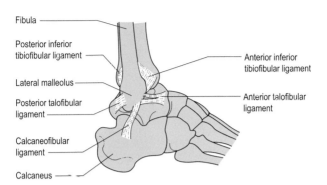

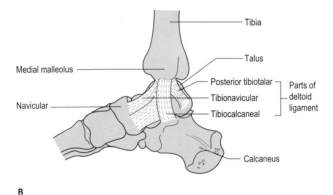

B

Figure 1.18, cont'd (B) Ankle ligaments. The lateral ligament runs from the lateral malleolus to the calcaneus and talus (neck and lateral tubercle) bones. The medial ligament runs from the medial malleolus to the navicular (tuberosity), calcaneus (anterior-medial margin of sustentaculum tali) and talus (medial tubercle) bones.

The foot joints:

● Include the:
— subtalar joint where eversion and inversion occur
— midtarsal joints (talocalcaneonavicular and calcaneocuboidal) where eversion and inversion occur
— tarsometatarsal, intermetatarsal, metatarsophalangeal and interphalangeal joints.

- Are all synovial joints except the fibrous cuboidonavicular joint.

MUSCLES (Figure 1.16)

The leg has a robust interosseous membrane that connects the tibia and fibula with anterior, lateral and posterior compartments divided by strong intermuscular septa.

- Anterior compartment (tibialis anterior, extensor digitorum longus, extensor hallucis longus, peroneus tertius):
  — is innervated by the deep peroneal nerve
  — is responsible for toe extension, foot dorsiflexion and contributions to foot inversion (tibialis anterior) and eversion (peroneus tertius) (Table 1.8).
- Lateral compartment (peroneus brevis, peroneus longus):
  — is innervated by the superficial peroneal nerve
  — is responsible for foot eversion and plantarflexion (Table 1.8).
- Posterior compartment (gastrocnemius, plantaris, soleus, tibialis posterior, flexor digitorum longus, flexor hallucis longus):
  — is innervated by the tibial nerve
  — is responsible for plantarflexion, toe flexion and foot inversion (tibialis posterior) (Tables 1.8 and 1.9)
  — gastrocnemius and plantaris provide minor contributions to knee flexion.

The intrinsic muscles of the foot are divided into four layers. They are responsible for the movements of the toes (Table 1.9).

BLOOD SUPPLY

- The anterior tibial artery supplies the anterior compartment of the leg and the ankle joint:
  — the origin is the popliteal artery and it starts at the inferior edge of the popliteus muscle
  — it is susceptible to ischaemia due to anterior compartment syndrome
  — it becomes the dorsalis pedis artery (palpable between extensor hallucis longus medially and extensor digitorum longus laterally) as it passes inferiorly to the extensor retinaculum anterior to the ankle, which supplies the foot and then forms the plantar arch (anastomosis with lateral

TABLE 1.8 The muscles, with their innervations, which provide movement at the ankle joint and foot (eversion and inversion)

Movement	Muscle	Origin	Insertion	Nerve
Dorsiflexion	Extensor hallucis longus (A)	Fibula and interosseous membrane	Big toe, distal phalanx	Deep peroneal
	Extensor digitorum longus (A)	Tibia and interosseous membrane	Middle/distal phalanx (lateral 4 toes)	Deep peroneal
	Peroneus tertius (A)	Fibula and interosseous membrane	5th MT base	Deep peroneal
	Tibialis anterior (A)	Tibia and interosseous membrane	1st MT base, medial cuneiform	Deep peroneal
Plantarflexion	Peroneus longus (L)	Fibula	1st MT, medial cuneiform	Superficial peroneal
	Peroneus brevis (L)	Fibula	5th MT	Superficial peroneal
	Plantaris (PS)	Lateral supracondyle of femur	Calcaneum	Tibial
	Gastrocnemius (PS)	Posterior condyles of femur	Calcaneum (via AT)	Tibial
	Soleus (PS)	Fibula and medial border of tibia	Calcaneum (via AT)	Ticial
	Flexor digitorum longus (PD)	Posterior aspect of tibia	Distal phalanges (lateral 4 toes)	Tibial
	Flexor hallucis longus (PD)	Posterior aspect of fibula	Distal phalanx of big toe	Tibial
	Tibialis posterior (PD)	Tibia and fibula	Navicular, medial cuneiform	Tibial
Eversion	Peroneus tertius (A)	Anterior aspect of fibula	5th MT base	Deep peroneal
	Peroneus lorgus (L)	Fibula	1st MT, medial cuneiform	Superficial peroneal
	Peroneus brevis (L)	Fibula	5th MT	Superficial peroneal
Inversion	Tibialis anterior (A)	Tibia and interosseous membrane	1st MT base, medial cuneiform	Deep peroneal
	Tibialis posterior (PD)	Tibia and fibula	Navicular, medial cuneiform	Tibial

A, anterior compartment of leg; AT, Achilles' tendon; D, deep; L, lateral compartment of leg; MT, metatarsal; P, posterior compartment of leg; S, superficial.

TABLE 1.9 The muscles, with their innervations, which provide movement of the toes

Movement	Muscle	Origin	Insertion	Nerve
Big toe abduction	Abductor hallucis (1st layer)	Calcaneum, FR, PA	Big toe, proximal phalanx	Medial plantar
Big toe adduction	Adductor hallucis (3rd layer) Oblique head Transverse head	2nd → 4th MT bases Transverse ligament	Big toe, proximal phalanx Big toe, proximal phalanx	Lateral plantar
Big toe flexion	Flexor hallucis longus Flexor hallucis brevis (3rd layer)	Posterior aspect of fibula Cuboid, cuneiforms	Big toe, distal phalanx Big toe, proximal phalanx	Tibial Medial plantar
Big toe extension	Extensor hallucis longus	Fibula and interosseous membrane	Big toe, distal phalanx	Deep peroneal
Little toe abduction	Abductor digiti minimi (1st layer)	Calcaneus, PA	5th toe, proximal phalanx	Lateral plantar
Little toe flexion	Flexor digiti minimi brevis (3rd layer)	5th MT	5th toe, proximal phalanx	Medial plantar
Digital abduction	Dorsal interossei (4th layer)	MT	Digits, proximal phalanx	Lateral plantar
Digital adduction	Plantar interossei (4th layer)	3rd–5th MT	Digits, proximal phalanx	Lateral plantar
Digital flexion	Flexor digitorum longus Flexor digitorum brevis (1st layer)	Posterior aspect of tibia Calcaneum, PA	Distal phalanx (lateral 4 toes) Middle phalanx (lateral 4 toes)	Tibial Medial plantar
Digital extension	Extensor digitorum longus	Tibia and interosseous membrane	Middle/distal phalanx (lateral 4 toes)	Deep peroneal

FR, flexor retinaculum; MT, metatarsal; PA, plantar aponeurosis. The lumbricals are responsible for PIPJ flexion and IPJ/DIPJ extension.

plantar artery), which gives rise to metatarsal and digital arteries.

- The posterior tibial artery supplies the posterior and lateral compartments of the leg and the ankle joint:
  — the origin is the popliteal artery and it starts at the inferior edge of the popliteus muscle
  — it runs inferior to soleus and gastrocnemius
  — it gives rise to the peroneal (fibular) artery ~2–3 cm below popliteus that predominantly supplies the lateral compartment of the leg
  — it becomes the medial and lateral plantar arteries (as it passes inferiorly to the flexor retinaculum), which supply the foot via their own branches and the palmar arch.

NERVES

- The common peroneal nerve (L4–L5, S1–S2) arises after a division of the sciatic nerve just superior to the popliteal fossa (lateral to the tibial nerve), where it provides some innervation to the knee joint. It then circles the fibula neck and divides to give:
  — sensory cutaneous divisions (sural nerve)
  — the deep peroneal nerve (passes inferiorly to the extensor retinaculum), which innervates the ankle joint and the anterior compartment of the leg, and provides sensation to the 1st web space of the dorsum of the foot (Figure 1.19)
  — the superficial peroneal nerve, which innervates the lateral compartment of the leg and some intrinsic muscles of the foot, and provides sensation to the anterior aspect of the leg and the dorsum of the foot (Figure 1.19).

- The tibial nerve (L4–L5, S1–S3) arises after a division of the sciatic nerve just superior to the popliteal fossa (superficial to popliteal vessels). It innervates the posterior compartment of the leg (runs inferiorly to the soleus) as well as the ankle joint. The nerve passes posterior to the medial malleolus and then divides as it passes inferiorly to the flexor retinaculum to give:
  — the medial and lateral plantar nerves, which innervate the intrinsic muscles of the foot and provide sensory innervation to the sole of the foot (Figure 1.19)
  — sensory cutaneous divisions (sural nerve).

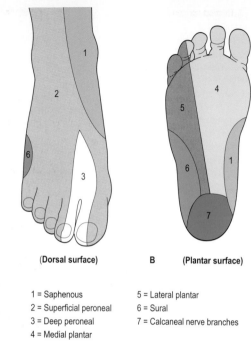

A (Dorsal surface)   **B** (Plantar surface)

1 = Saphenous   5 = Lateral plantar
2 = Superficial peroneal 6 = Sural
3 = Deep peroneal   7 = Calcaneal nerve branches
4 = Medial plantar

Figure 1.19 Sensory innervation of the foot: (A) dorsal; (B) plantar.

- The sural cutaneous nerve (derived from the tibial and common peroneal nerves) provides sensory innervation to the posterior and lateral aspects of the leg, as well as the lateral aspect of the plantar and dorsal parts of the foot (Figure 1.19)
- The saphenous nerve originates from the femoral nerve and provides sensory innervation to the medial aspect of the leg and ankle (Figure 1.19).

SPINE

BONES AND JOINTS (Figures 1.20 and 1.21)

The vertebral column begins with the cervical vertebrae below the skull (atlanto-occipital joint), ending with the fused vertebrae that

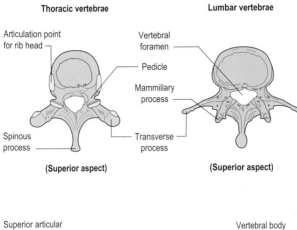

Thoracic vertebrae

Lumbar vertebrae

Articulation point for rib head

Vertebral foramen

Pedicle

Mammillary process

Spinous process

Transverse process

(Superior aspect)

(Superior aspect)

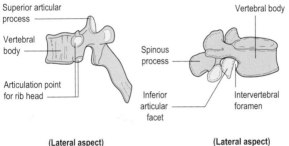

Superior articular process

Vertebral body

Articulation point for rib head

Spinous process

Inferior articular facet

Vertebral body

Intervertebral foramen

(Lateral aspect)

(Lateral aspect)

Figure 1.20 Characteristic features of individual vertebrae. The synovial articular facet joints provide articulation between the individual vertebrae. These joints are supported by surrounding ligaments (supra- and interspinous, anterior and posterior longitudinal, and ligamenta flava).

form the sacrum and the coccyx. The primary curvatures are found in the thoracic and sacrococcygeal regions. The secondary curvatures are found in the cervical and lumbar regions. Most vertebrae have an anterior body and a posterior ring (pedicle, lamina, lateral and posterior spinous processes) which protect nervous elements within the spinal canal. They are separated by the intervertebral disc consisting of a nucleus pulposus within an annulus fibrosus. Longitudinal ligaments also add to intervertebral strength.

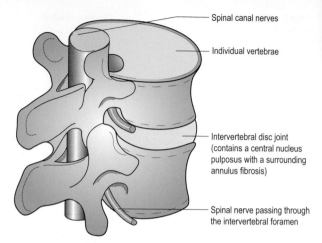

Spinal canal nerves

Individual vertebrae

Intervertebral disc joint (contains a central nucleus pulposus with a surrounding annulus fibrosis)

Spinal nerve passing through the intervertebral foramen

Figure 1.21 The secondary cartilaginous intervertebral disc (consists of the nucleus pulposus and annulus fibrosus) joint provides the macro movements of the spine. With increasing years the nucleus pulposus will dry out (which can lead to back pain) and herniate through the annulus fibrosus (a slipped disc). This can in turn lead to compression of the nerve roots, which may lead to pain and paraesthesia down the leg (sciatica).

MUSCLES OF THE THORACOLUMBAR GROUP (Figure 1.22)

● Extrinsic muscles of the back involve those connected with movement of the shoulder and arm (e.g. latissimus dorsi) and those connected with breathing (e.g. serratus posterior)
● The intrinsic muscles of the back are those involved with the fundamental movements of the spine (e.g. erector spinae, quadratus lumborum, psoas major). Unbalanced muscle action can lead to displacement and rotation of a section of the vertebrae, i.e. scoliosis.

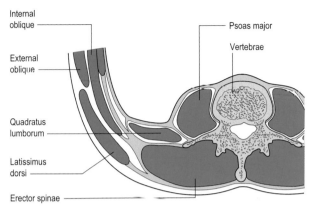

Figure 1.22 Muscles of the back. The erector spinae muscles are involved in spinal flexion and extension, as well as lateral flexion. The transversospinalis muscles are involved in spinal extension and rotation. The intertransversarii and interspinales muscles are involved in spinal extension and lateral flexion.

BLOOD SUPPLY

The blood supply of the vertebral column comprises:

- Cervical, e.g. vertebral or basilar arteries
- Thoracic, e.g. intercostal or anterior spinal arteries
- Lumbar, e.g. lumbar segmental or common iliac arteries
- Sacral, e.g. internal iliac or sacral arteries.

CHAPTER 2

HISTORY AND EXAMINATION

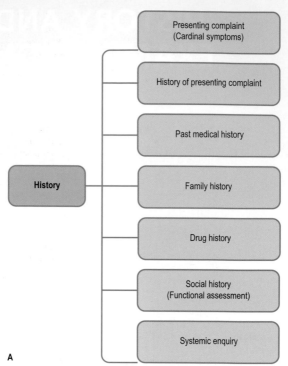

Figure 2.1 The algorithm for history (**A**) and examination (**B**) of the musculoskeletal system. When examining, the headings Inspect, Feel, Move and Special tests comprise a logical order worth remembering.

HISTORY TAKING

PRESENTING COMPLAINT

This should be a simple description of the problem, e.g. injured left ankle, painful left hip.

HISTORY OF PRESENTING COMPLAINT

Ask the patient to recall the onset of the primary symptoms and their nature:

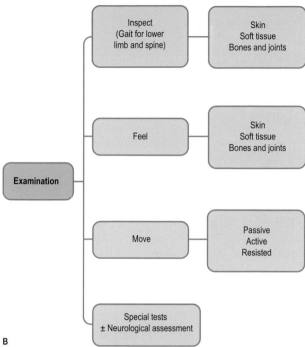

B

Figure 2.1, cont'd Please see the inner cover for details of the neurological assessment of the upper and lower limb.

- Acute vs. chronic
- Monoarticular vs. oligo/polyarticular
- Small vs. large joints
- Precipitating factors, e.g. medications, trauma.

Remember to cover the cardinal symptoms of the musculoskeletal system:

- Pain (joint or bone):
  — SOCRATES: **S**ite, **O**nset, **C**haracter, **R**adiation, **A**lleviating factors, **T**iming, **E**xacerbating factors, **S**everity.
- Swelling, redness and heat:
  — SOCRATES.
- Loss of function:
  — effect on activities of daily living.
- Weakness

● Red flag symptoms are important to exclude if any sinister diagnosis is contemplated.

PAST MEDICAL HISTORY

It is key to enquire about previously diagnosed rheumatological disorders, e.g. rheumatoid, vasculitides, osteoarthritis, osteoporosis. Similarly, it is important to determine if there have been any episodes of trauma in the past, including operations, e.g. previous ACL rupture, total hip replacement. Fundamental co-morbidities to enquire about are:

● Ischaemic heart disease
● Diabetes and other endocrine disorders, e.g. hypothyroidism
● Chronic obstructive airways disease or asthma
● Epilepsy
● Previous PE/DVT
● Chronic kidney disease
● HIV/AIDS, e.g. immunosuppression is a risk factor for septic arthritis.

FAMILY HISTORY

Common musculoskeletal disorders that may present with a significant family history are:

● Inflammatory arthropathies, e.g. RA
● Seronegative arthritides (ankylosing spondylitis, reactive arthritis, psoriatic arthritis)
● Gout
● Hypermobility syndrome
● Connective tissue disorders
● Congenital abnormalities, e.g. developmental dysplasia of the hip.
● Some primary bone tumours

DRUG HISTORY (see Chapter 8)

Important medications to enquire about are:

● Analgesia:
 — NSAIDs due to potential side effects, e.g. GI bleed, renal impairment

  — opiates due to potential side effects and tolerance; also a
  useful marker of pain severity in most cases.
- Steroids, as long-term use predisposes to osteoporosis, along
  with numerous other side effects
- Diuretics, particularly thiazides, are common precipitants in
  gout
- Minocycline, hydralazine and procainamide are potential
  precipitants of drug-induced lupus
- DMARDs due to the large number of potential side effects,
  e.g. immunosuppression
- Over-the-counter medications
- Drug allergies.

SOCIAL HISTORY

A full functional assessment should be performed, including:

- Occupation, including partner's
- Family dynamics:
  - Is there a disabled elderly parent or spouse to look
    after?
  - What about children? Are they nearby to help if an
    operation with prolonged recovery is contemplated?
- Activities of daily living, e.g. washing, dressing, walking
  (stairs), writing, meal preparation
- Alcohol consumption
- Smoking and recreational drugs
- Diet.

SYSTEMIC ENQUIRY

This should cover the areas of common extra-articular
features:

- Systemic upset, e.g. fevers, sweats
- Nails, e.g. pitting
- Skin, e.g. rash
- Eyes, e.g. red, dry, painful.

It is also important to cover the standard systemic enquiry
covering the cardiovascular, respiratory, gastrointestinal,
genitourinary and neurological systems.

WRIST AND HAND

INSPECT

- Skin and nail alterations:
  - onycholysis and pitting in psoriatic patients
  - nail infarcts and ulcers in vasculitis
  - palmar erythema.
- Muscle wasting (note if unilateral or diffuse):
  - thenar eminence (e.g. median nerve compression in carpal tunnel syndrome)
  - hypothenar eminence (ulnar nerve injury)
  - interosseous muscles (intermetacarpal recession on dorsum of hand sometimes seen in RA).
- Swelling, redness and heat:
  - joints (RA, OA, infection)
  - tendons and tendon sheaths (RA, infection).
- Deformities:
  - subluxations and fractures
  - swan neck, boutonnière, nodules, ulnar deviation, Z-thumb deformity in RA (see Chapter 5)
  - Heberden's nodes and Bouchard's nodes in OA (see Chapter 5)
  - tophi (gout and pseudogout)
  - sclerodactyly (diabetes, scleroderma, SLE)
  - thickening of the palmar fascia (Dupuytren's contracture).

FEEL

- Joint and soft tissue tenderness e.g. anatomical snuff box
- Swelling and temperature of bone or soft tissue
- Flexor tendon (sheaths) for swelling and thickening
- Sensation over the ulnar, radial and median nerve innervations (see Figure 1.12)
- Crepitus and trigger finger on joint movement.

MOVE

- Ask if any pain on movement
- Pinch strength, precision pinch and grip strength
- Wrist radial deviation 0–25°, ulnar deviation 0–50°, dorsiflexion 0–90° (Figure 2.2) and palmarflexion 0–90° (Figure 2.3)

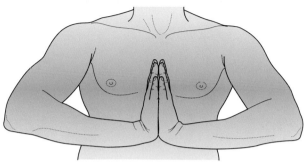

Figure 2.2 Wrist dorsiflexion (the prayer sign).

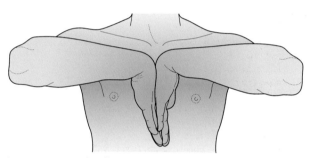

Figure 2.3 Wrist palmarflexion.

- MCP, PIP and DIP joint flexion and extension
- Specific muscles and/or nerves:
  — abductor pollicis brevis (median nerve): thumb abduction
  — adductor pollicis (ulnar nerve): thumb adduction (Froment's sign, Figure 2.4)
  — flexor pollicis longus (median nerve): thumb IPJ flexion
  — flexor pollicis brevis: thumb MCPJ flexion
  — extensor pollicis longus and extensor pollicis brevis (C7 radial nerve): thumb IPJ and MCPJ extension (respectively)
  — dorsal and palmar interossei (ulnar nerve): finger abduction and adduction, respectively
  — flexor digitorum profundus (median and ulnar nerve): DIPJ flexion (hold PIPJ in fixed extension)
  — flexor digitorum superficialis (median nerve): PIPJ flexion (hold all other fingers in fixed extension).

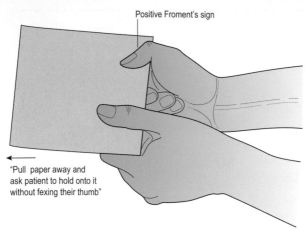

Positive Froment's sign

←
"Pull paper away and
ask patient to hold onto it
without fexing their thumb"

Figure 2.4 Froment's sign. The patient cannot hold onto the paper
without flexion of the right thumb IPJ due to a weakness of right thumb
adduction.

SPECIAL TESTS

- Finkelstein's test (De Quervain's tenosynovitis, see
  Chapter 4)
- Tinel's and Phalen's tests (carpal tunnel syndrome, see
  Chapter 4).

ELBOW AND FOREARM

INSPECT

- Swelling, redness and heat:
  — olecranon bursitis (RA)
  — psoriatic plaques on extensor surfaces
  — effusion (often found in the lateral infracondylar space).
- Deformities:
  — joints (RA, OA, infection)
  — tendons and tendon sheaths (RA)
  — fracture and/or dislocation
  — disturbance of normal carrying angle, i.e. cubitus varus
    after supracondylar fractures
  — muscle wasting.

FEEL

- Regional tenderness or temperature:
  — epicondyles (golfer's and tennis elbow, ulnar irritation).
- Olecranon:
  — nodules (RA), effusion, tophi.
- Crepitus on joint movement, including radial head on supination and pronation.

MOVE

- Ask if any pain on movement
- Flexion and extension (0–150°)
- Pronation (0–90°) and supination (0–90°) with elbows flexed to 90° and shoulders adducted
- Collateral ligaments with arm in extension.

SHOULDER

INSPECT

- Anterior and posterior:
  — shoulder contour symmetry.
- Muscle wasting:
  — frozen shoulder
  — rotator cuff pathology.
- Swelling, redness and heat:
  — effusion; may be hidden by deltoid muscle.
- Deformities:
  — scapula winging (e.g. long thoracic nerve palsy)
  — shoulder dislocation (ACJ or glenohumeral 'step')
  — prominent acromioclavicular or sternoclavicular joint.

FEEL

- Joint and soft tissue tenderness and/or swelling at the:
  — acromioclavicular, sternoclavicular, glenohumeral joints
  — clavicle (check if unstable)
  — shoulder point and subacromial space
  — scapular spine.
- Crepitus on joint movement.
- Sensation over the axillary nerve cutaneous innervation (regimental patch sign).

MOVE

- Ask if any pain on movement
- Hands behind head, push elbows back (Figure 2.5A):
  — checks shoulder flexion, abduction and external (lateral) rotation.
- Hands together behind back (Figure 2.5B):
  — checks shoulder extension, adduction and internal (medial) rotation.
- Specific movements of the shoulder joint:
  — medial and lateral rotation (range 180°) with the elbow flexed to 90° and the shoulder in full adduction (Figure 2.6A)

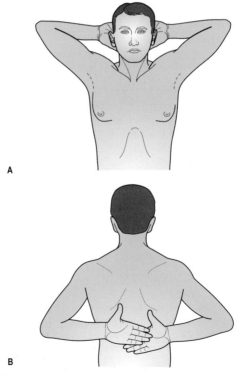

A

B

Figure 2.5 For an impression of shoulder movements. (A) Hands behind head with elbows pushed back. (B) Hands behind back with elbows pushed back. (Adapted from Ford et al 2005.)

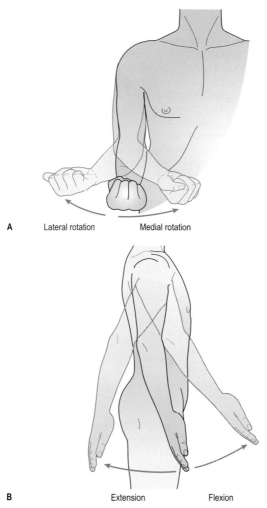

A   Lateral rotation   Medial rotation

B   Extension   Flexion

Figure 2.6 Movements of the shoulder joint. (A) Lateral and medial rotation of the shoulder. Lateral rotation is lost early in **frozen shoulder**. Pain on resisted lateral (external) rotation is indicative of infraspinatus pathology. Pain on resisted medial (internal) rotation is indicative of subscapularis pathology. (B) Flexion and extension of the shoulder. (Adapted from Ford et al 2005.)

— flexion (180°) and extension (60°) using a hand on the blade of the scapula to immobilize it (Figure 2.6B)
— abduction (180°) and adduction (30°) using a hand on the blade of the scapula to immobilize it (Figure 2.7). 0–90° of abduction is due to the glenohumeral joint alone, whereas after 90° the glenohumeral joint and scapula are both responsible for abduction.

- Rotator cuff:
  — painful abduction against resistance = supraspinatus tendon inflammation
  — active initiation possible, pain between 40 and 120° = painful arc syndrome (Figure 2.8) which is seen in rotator cuff impingement; symptoms reproduced when shoulder abducted to ~100° and internally rotated (Hawkin's Test for supraspinatus impingement)
  — passive abduction to 45°, active abduction thereafter (due to deltoid) = rotator cuff (supraspinatus) rupture
  — pain on resisted medial rotation = subscapularis pathology (Gerber's Test to confirm)
  — pain on resisted lateral rotation = infraspinatus pathology.

SPECIAL TESTS

- Brachial plexus assessment
  — motor and sensory assessment can be guided using the tables and diagram on the inner cover.
- Yergason's test
  — forearm supination against resistance indicative of biceps tendon inflammation.
- Scapular winging test
  — push against wall, scapula becomes prominent medial winging – injury of long thoracic nerve (C5–C7) e.g. during lymph node resection in axilla
  — lateral winging – trapezius weakness (accessory spinal nerve).

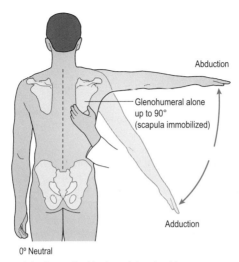

Figure 2.7 Abduction and adduction of the shoulder.

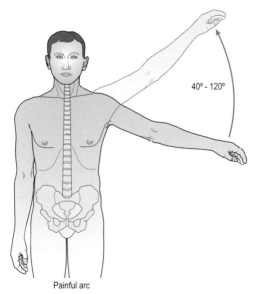

Figure 2.8 Painful arc syndrome is indicative of subacromial impingement. A painful arc towards 160–180° is indicative of acromioclavicular pathology. (Adapted from Ford et al 2005.)

HIP

INSPECT

- Gait to look at rhythm and symmetry:
  - Trendelenburg (waddling or rolling) gait is due to a dysfunction of the pelvic abductors, thus not raising the pelvis on the weight-bearing side when walking
  - Trendelenburg's test (Figure 2.9) may be positive with weak gluteal abductors e.g. DDH, coxa vara, polio, hip dislocation or femoral neck deformities
  - antalgic gait is a pain-reducing gait as the patient attempts to decrease weight bearing on the affected hip, e.g. a short-stride gait so as to reduce the time spent on the painful hip
  - drop foot gait is due to weak dorsiflexor muscles of the ankle, e.g. in a common peroneal neuropathy. Gait involves a high-stepping knee with toe planting.
- Standing:
  - scoliosis, kyphosis, loss of lumbar lordosis in muscle spasm.
- Supine:
  - check pelvis at right angles to spine
  - swelling (effusion), redness, heat, muscle wasting e.g. gluteal, deformity, surgical scars
  - FFD using Thomas' test: patient supine, place hand under lumbar lordosis and flex the unaffected normal hip. The lordosis will flatten onto your hand and FFD of the affected hip becomes apparent.

FEEL

- Joint, bone and soft tissue tenderness or swelling:
  - pelvis (e.g. ASIS and PSIS) and greater trochanter (bursitis).
- Leg length measured with legs flat and in same abduction angle (Figure 2.10):
  - true: anterior superior iliac spine to medial malleolus
  - apparent: xiphisternum to medial malleolus
  - Galleazzi test confirms discrepancy at either tibia or femur.

MOVE

- Ask if any pain on movement
- Hip flexion 0–120° (supine) and extension 20° (prone)

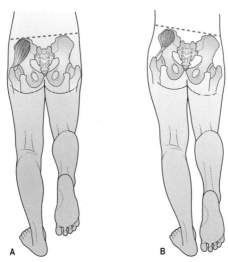

Figure 2.9 Trendelenburg's test. Kneel down in front of the patient with your hands on their anterior superior iliac spines. Request the patient to lift each leg in turn by bending it at the knee, thus weight bearing on one leg. (A) Normal abductor function of the left leg, so as the left side of the pelvis lowers the right rises. (B) Deficient abductor function of the left leg, so the left side of the pelvis rises and the right lowers.

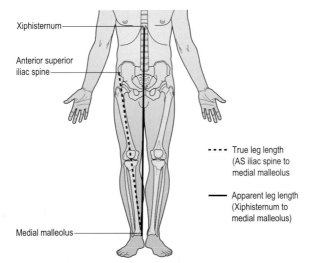

Figure 2.10 True and apparent leg length measurement. (Adapted from Ford et al 2005.)

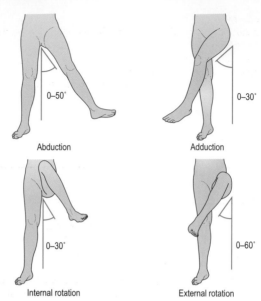

0–50°

Abduction

0–30°

Adduction

0–30°

Internal rotation

0–60°

External rotation

Figure 2.11 Hip abduction and adduction. Hip external and internal rotation. Decreased abduction and internal rotation can be indicative of OA of the hip. (Adapted from Ford et al 2005.)

- Patient and pelvis stabilized by placing arm over contralateral anterior superior iliac spine:
  — abduction 0–50°, adduction 0–30° (Figure 2.11).
- Patient supine with hip and knee flexed to 90°:
  — internal rotation 0–30°, external rotation 0–60° (Figure 2.11).

KNEE

INSPECT

- Gait and standing deformities:
  — fixed flexion deformity
  — valgus (distance between medial malleoli i.e. genu valgum)
  — varus (distance between medial condyles of femur i.e. genu varum).

- Muscle wasting:
  — quadriceps: if notable, measure left and right quad thickness 10 cm above each patella.
- Swelling, redness and heat:
  — anterior and posterior inspection
  — anterior effusion (horseshoe shape) superior to knee
  — surgical scars.
- Supine deformities:
  — bony contours
  — knee alignment.

FEEL

- Joint line and ligament tenderness (with knee flexed 45°)
- Swelling:
  — posteriorly in the popliteal fossa (Baker's cyst)
  — prepatellar bursitis (housemaid's knee)
  — infrapatellar bursitis (clergyman's knee).
- Effusion:
  — massage (cross-fluctuation) test: knee extended, massage upwards on the medial aspect of the knee to remove fluid from the anteromedial compartment, then massage down the lateral aspect of the knee and observe as fluid is displaced back into the compartment
  — patellar tap (Figure 2.12): knee extended, remove fluid from the suprapatellar pouch as shown, then push down on the patella and a palpable 'tap' should be felt.
- Crepitus on joint movement
- Redness and/or heat.

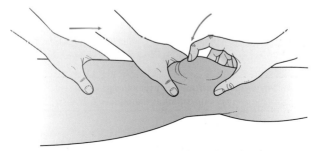

Figure 2.12 Testing for an effusion using the patellar tap test. (Adapted from Ford et al 2005.)

MOVE

- Ask if any pain on movement
- Knee extension and flexion (0–140°, 15–140° if there is an FFD)
- Test cruciate and collateral ligaments (Figure 2.13)

SPECIAL TESTS

- Lachman's test is an alternative for ACL instability (knee flexed to 20°, one hand on thigh and one hand behind the tibia with the thumb on the tibial tuberosity, pull tibia anteriorly)
- McMurray's test for meniscal injury (click at the lateral joint line occurs while extending and internally/externally rotating the foot). Apley's is an alternative.
- Straight leg raise for extensor mechanism weakness and/or rupture (see Chapter 4).

ANKLE AND FOOT

INSPECT

- Gait and standing deformities:
  — hindfoot: varus or valgus
  — plantar arches: place hand in arch of foot, see if high (pes cavus) or low (pes planus)
  — toes: mallet, hammer, claw (Figure 2.14).
- Supine deformities:
  — nails: clubbing or pitting
  — skin: callosities, athletes foot
  — swelling, redness and heat: e.g. gout of the big toe
  — talipes equinovarus, hallux valgus (MTP joint abduction), hallux rigidus.

FEEL

- Joint and soft tissue tenderness, crepitus, heat and swelling:
  — forefoot (e.g. MTPJs), mid-foot (e.g. navicular) and hindfoot (e.g. malleoli, talus and Achilles).

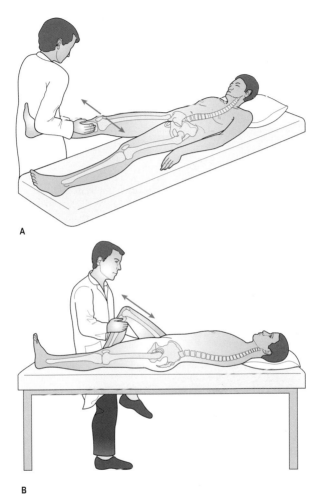

A

B

Figure 2.13 (A) The collateral ligaments are tested with the knee fully extended and the foot under the examiner's arm. Varus and valgus positional pressure on the knee tests the lateral and medial collateral ligaments. (B) The anterior draw test involves flexing the knee to 90° and pulling the tibia forward (ACL). The posterior draw test involves flexing the knee to 90° and pushing the tibia backwards (PCL). The examiner sits on the patient's foot with both hands placed on the flexed knee as shown in B. (Adapted from Ford et al 2005.)

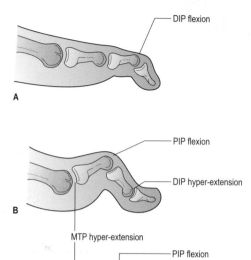

Figure 2.14 Deformities of the foot: (A) mallet toe; (B) hammer toe affects the middle toes most commonly; (C) claw toe due to weakness of the lumbrical and interosseous muscles. The latter two are associated with hallux valgus or poor-fitting shoes. Surgical intervention may be required if conservation treatment is ineffective. (Adapted from Coote & Haslam 2004.)

MOVE

- Dorsiflexion (0–10°) and plantarflexion (0–30°) (Figure 2.15)
- Inversion/supination (0–30°) and eversion/pronation (0–20°)
- Test subtalar joint movement:
  — stabilize ankle and move calcaneum inwards and outwards.
- Test midtarsal movement:
  — stabilize heel and invert and evert forefoot (midtarsal movements).

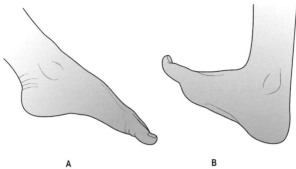

A   **B**

Figure 2.15 Ankle plantarflexion (A – push the accelerator) and dorsiflexion (B – release the accelerator). NB: Dorsiflexion is greater with the knee flexed due to relaxation of the gastrocnemius muscle. Pes planus is flattening of the medial longitudinal arch.

SPECIAL TESTS

- Thompson's or Simmon's test for calf squeeze test. (see Chapter 4):
  — patient supine and on their front with both feet hanging off the end of the bed
  — squeeze mid-calf region and look for plantarflexion
  — Achilles tendon rupture = no plantarflexion is seen
  — a step may be palpable where the rupture has occurred.
- Discriminate rigid (pathological) from flexible flat foot:
  — tiptoe stance
  — plantar arch should accentuate in flexible flat foot, and hindfoot moves into varus.

SPINE

INSPECT

- Muscle wasting
- Swelling, redness or heat
- Anteriorly, posteriorly and laterally for deformities (Figure 2.16):
  — scoliosis (see Chapter 4)
  — torticollis in the neck
  — kyphosis
  — lordosis.

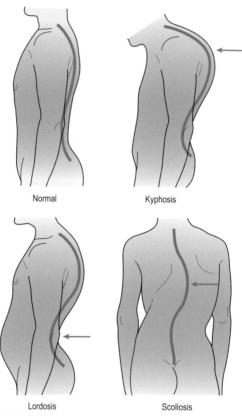

Normal

Kyphosis

Lordosis

Scoliosis

Figure 2.16 Possible appearances of posture on inspection. (Adapted from Ford et al 2005.)

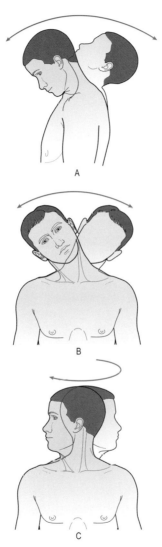

Figure 2.17 (A) Cervical flexion and extension. (B) Cervical lateral flexion. (C) Cervical rotation. (Adapted from Ford et al 2005.)

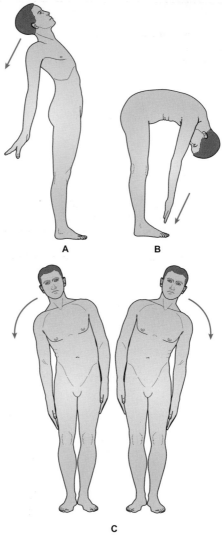

Figure 2.18 (A) Spine extension. (B) Spine flexion. (C) Spinal lateral flexion. (Adapted from Ford et al 2005.)

FEEL

- For tenderness, heat and swelling:
  — paraspinals
  — spine (processes)
  — bony contours
  — soft tissues.

MOVE

- Neck/cervical spine (Figure 2.17):
  — flexion (80°) and extension (60°)
  — rotation left and right (0–80°)
  — lateral flexion left and right (0–45°).
- Thoracic and lumbar spine (Figure 2.18):
  — flexion (touch your toes) and extension
  — rotation left and right of the thoracic spine (with patient sitting)
  — lateral flexion (slide left arm down left leg and vice versa).

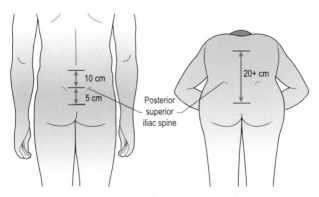

Figure 2.19 Schober's test. From the midline, two marks are placed 5 cm inferiorly and 10 cm superiorly to the level of the posterior superior iliac spines. During spinal flexion the superior mark should normally displace upwards ≥5 cm. Less than this would be an indication of pathology such as ankylosing spondylitis. (Adapted from Ford et al 2005.)

SPECIAL TESTS

- Schober's test (Figure 2.19)
- Sciatica (L4/L5 or L5/S1 disc prolapse):
  — with the patient supine and leg fully extended, raise leg from bed (straight leg raise). Pain and/or paraesthesiae present in back and leg if positive
  — Bragaard's test is positive when you dorsiflex the ankle during the straight leg raise; pain and/or paraesthesia are worse.
- Femoral nerve irritation (L2/L3 or L3/L4 disc prolapse):
  — with the patient prone and leg fully extended, raise leg from couch (femoral stretch test). Pain and/or paraesthesiae present in front of thigh if positive.

CHAPTER 3

INVESTIGATIONS

BASIC HAEMATOLOGICAL AND BIOCHEMICAL INVESTIGATIONS

FULL BLOOD COUNT (Table 3.1)

ESR and CRP

An increase in ESR (aggregation of erythrocytes) and/or CRP is indicative of inflammation and/or infection. CRP is more specific and rises within 10 hours of the onset of infection and inflammation. Changes in the ESR are slower, and there are other possible causes for a raised ESR including myeloproliferative disorders such as multiple myeloma. In these situations the CRP may be normal. An alternative measure of ESR is the plasma viscosity as it is also elevated during the inflammatory process.

The characteristic biochemical profile of an acute phase response is characterized by:

● Normochromic, normocytic anaemia
● Neutrophilia
● Thrombocytosis
● A raised CRP and ESR
● A decreased albumin level.

TABLE 3.1 The potential conditions associated with abnormalities of the full blood count differential

Analysis	Condition(s) indicated
Haemoglobin	
Normochromic normocytic anaemia	Acute/chronic inflammation, malignancy, autoimmune disease
Hypochromic microcytic anaemia	NSAID treatment may cause GI bleeding and iron deficiency anaemia
White cell count	
Neutrophilia	Bacterial infection/sepsis, steroids, systemic vasculitis
Neutropenia	Felty's syndrome, SLE, DMARD therapy
Lymphopenia	SLE, steroids, viral infection
Eosinophilia	Churg–Strauss syndrome
Platelets	
Thrombocytosis	Acute/chronic postoperative inflammation
Thrombocytopenia	DMARD therapy, Felty's syndrome, SLE, infection

Creatine kinase

Serum CK is measured in the investigation of muscle disease. It is a marker of muscle damage, with elevated levels of the different isoenzymes seen:

- CK-MM = motor neurone disease, muscular dystrophy, myositis, vasculitis, PE
- CK-MB = myocardial infarction
- Other, e.g. alcohol, drugs, excessive exercise, trauma, postoperatively, race (Afro-Caribbeans with high normal levels).

CK measurements are frequently used in conjunction with more specific tests such as electromyography or needle muscle biopsy for histology.

Urate, calcium biochemistry and liver function tests

Alterations in serum calcium, phosphate and alkaline phosphatase in bone disease are shown in Table 3.2. Uric acid levels are raised in gout but can be normal during the acute attack. Renal function may decline in connective tissue disorders, vasculitides and gout, with a rise in urea and creatinine seen. LFTs may be abnormal during flares of RA and in response to DMARD therapy (e.g. methotrexate, azathioprine).

Specialized markers of bone turnover

Urine (or serum) pyridinium crosslinks are formed from the breakdown of bone collagen during the process of bone remodelling and are therefore a marker of bone resorption. Osteocalcin is produced by osteoblasts during matrix deposition in the course of bone formation. These tests are not routinely available in most centres but are markers for increased bone resorption and formation.

IMMUNOLOGICAL TESTS

RHEUMATOID FACTOR (RF)

A strongly positive rheumatoid factor is typical of RA but is also found in other diseases:

- Sjögren's syndrome
- Systemic sclerosis
- SLE.

TABLE 3.2 The biochemical derangements associated with common bone disease and bony metastases

	Serum Ca^{2+}	Serum PO_4^-	Serum ALP	Serum PTH	Serum 25(OH)D
Osteoporosis	N	N	N	N	N
Paget's disease	N	N	↑	N	N
Osteomalacia	↓	↓	↑	↑	↓
Renal osteodystrophy	↓	↑	↑	↑↑	N
Primary hyperparathyroidism	↑	N/↓	N/↑	↑	N
Bone secondaries	↑	↑	↑	N	N

↑, increased; ↓, decreased; N, within normal range.
Adapted from Haslet et al (2002).

A weakly positive rheumatoid factor can also be found in:

- Chronic infection, e.g. hepatitis (viral), tuberculosis, endocarditis
- Hyperglobulinaemias, e.g. chronic liver disease
- Malignancy
- Elderly.

RF therefore has a low specificity for RA and a negative result does not exclude the diagnosis. It is a prognostic marker to some extent since high levels of RF are associated with more severe disease and nodules.

The methods of detection are based on the fact that RF is an antibody (commonly IgM anti-IgG) against the Fc portion of human IgG. The most popular detection technique employed is to add human IgG-coated latex beads to the patient's serum (Rose-Waaler test). The sheep-cell agglutination test is an alternative.

ANTI-CYCLIC CITRULLINATED PEPTIDE ANTIBODIES (ANTI-CCP)

Antibodies to CCPs have a high specificity for the diagnosis of RA (>95%) and can be present for months or years before the disease presents clinically. However, the sensitivity is relatively low since the CCP test may be negative in 30–40% of patients with a clinical diagnosis of RA. The usual method of detection is ELISA.

ANTINUCLEAR ANTIBODY (ANA)

A positive ANA is found in the following order of incidence:

- Drug-induced lupus (high specificity)
- SLE
- Systemic sclerosis
- Sjögren's syndrome
- Rheumatoid arthritis.

A weakly positive ANA can also be found in patients with:

- Autoimmune disease, e.g. chronic hepatitis, thyroid disorders
- Myasthenia gravis
- Widespread burns.

ANA is an autoantibody that targets a constituent of the nucleus, i.e. antibodies to nuclear antigens. As with RF, the clinical significance of ANA increases as the titre of antibodies increases. In the case of lupus, it is a useful diagnostic tool but not completely specific. The methods of detection involve indirect immunofluorescence microscopy using either rodent tissue substrate or human cell lines such as Hep-2.

ANTI-DNA ANTIBODY (dsDNA)

Anti-dsDNA is an autoantibody that targets double-stranded DNA. Raised levels have high specificity for acute SLE. A high value for IgG anti-dsDNA is an unfavourable prognostic marker specific to SLE.

ANTINEUTROPHIL CYTOPLASMIC ANTIBODY (ANCA)

ANCAs are antibodies that target neutrophil enzymes. Two patterns are common:

- PR3-ANCA (cytoplasmic) – associated with Wegener's granulomatosis
- MPO-ANCA (perinuclear) – associated with other vasculitides, e.g. PAN.

A positive MPO-ANCA can also be found in patients with IBD or a neoplasm.

JOINT ASPIRATION AND SYNOVIAL FLUID ANALYSIS

Acute or chronic non-infective monoarthritis associated with erythematous change is the primary indication for joint aspiration and fluid analysis as the character of the aspirate is suggestive of the degree of inflammation. It is the investigation of choice in:

- Crystal arthritis
- Reactive arthritis
- Intra-articular bleeding
- Trauma with an associated effusion
- Septic arthritis.

TABLE 3.3 Characteristics of inflammatory and non-inflammatory synovial fluid*

	Non-inflammatory synovial aspirate	Inflammatory synovial aspirate
Volume	Small	Large
Cell number	Low	High (leading to turbidity)
Appearance	Clear and colourless/pale yellow	Cloudy, translucent or opaque fluid with pus (pyarthrosis related to neutrophilia) and/or blood staining (haemarthrosis)
Viscosity	High due to hyaluronate	Low due to breakdown of hyaluronate

*A deposit of lipid superior to a haemarthrosis (severe synovitis, trauma or thrombophilia) is indicative of an intra-articular fracture.

Relative contraindications are:

- Potential for uncontrolled bleeding, e.g. a high INR
- Periarticular soft tissue or skin infection
- Joint replacement.

Potential complications are:

- Infection
- Bleeding
- Further effusion.

As the severity of joint inflammation increases (OA < RA < seronegative arthritis < crystal arthritis < septic arthritis), the synovial fluid takes on the characteristics shown in Table 3.3.

FOLLOW-UP INVESTIGATIONS

Gram staining and culture

Suspected sepsis means synovial fluid should be sent urgently to microbiology with antibiotic sensitivities requested. Common organisms are Gram-positive cocci, particularly staphylococci. These organisms, commonly sourced from the patient's skin or blood, are often indicated with prosthetic joint implant infection. Less common organisms are streptococci, TB, gonococcus, Gram-negative bacteria and anaerobes.

Polarized light microscopy compensated with red filter

This is performed if there is a suspected high crystal (urate or cholesterol) concentration due to white synovial fluid, to identify the crystals. Common results are:

- **Gout:** long, needle-shaped sodium urate crystals, with strong light intensity and negative birefringence
- **Pseudogout:** small rhomboid or rod-shaped calcium pyrophosphate crystals, commonly fewer in number, with weak light intensity and positive birefringence.

RADIOLOGY

Radiographs are still an essential diagnostic tool within rheumatology and orthopaedics. The following should be looked for on a bone radiograph:

- General: name, age, date of film, view, part of body, adequacy of film
- Soft tissues: wasting, swelling, calcification, free air
- Bones: fracture and classification (see Chapter 7), deformity, cyst, calcification, change in density
- Joints: joint space, erosions, calcification, sclerosis, new bone formation.

The **Ottawa Ankle Rules** state radiographs are indicated if there is:

- Inability to weight-bear immediately and/or four steps in the emergency department
- Bony tenderness along the distal 6 cm of the posterior edge or tip of the medial malleolus
- Bony tenderness along the distal 6 cm of the posterior edge or tip of the lateral malleolus
- Bony tenderness at the base of the navicular or fifth metatarsal bone in foot injuries, which require a foot radiograph.

The **Ottawa Knee Rules** state radiographs are required if there is:

- Age 55 or over
- Inability to weight-bear immediately and/or four steps in the emergency department
- Inability to flex to 90°

- Bony tenderness over the fibula head
- Isolated bony tenderness of the patella.

For details on interpreting children's radiographs, see Chapter 6.

OTHER IMAGING TECHNIQUES

BONE SCINTIGRAPHY (ISOTOPE BONE SCAN)

Using gamma-camera imaging and i.v. radionuclides, e.g. ^{99m}Tc-bisphosphonate, bone scintigraphy is a useful, and powerful, imaging technique. Increased uptake of the radionuclide reflects vascularization and bone formation. Uptake is increased in conditions associated with increased bone turnover and uptake is decreased in avascular bone. Isotope bone scans are useful in defining the extent of Paget's disease and in the diagnosis of bone metastases. Depending on when the images are viewed postinjection, it is possible to use the highly sensitive bone scanning technique for multiple, although non-specific, diagnostic purposes:

- Early (seconds):
  — bone vascularity
  — inflammation, e.g. synovitis
  — bone or joint infection
  — bone tumours.
- Late (hours):
  — bone remodelling and abnormal bone turnover, e.g. in a stress fracture.

DUAL ENERGY X-RAY ABSORPTIOMETRY (DEXA)

DEXA is a measure of BMD and is used in the investigation and management of osteoporosis. The risk factors for osteoporosis are indications for this test (see Chapter 5).

The principle of DEXA is shown in Figure 3.1. Scanning is most often preferred at the hip and spine. Along with a BMD value, most scanners will give:

- Z-score: number of standard deviations the BMD deviates from the population average for the age of the patient

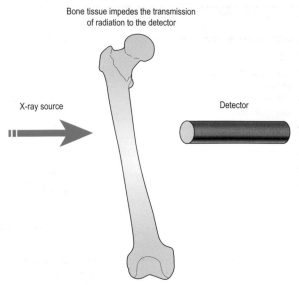

Figure 3.1 The principle of DEXA scanning. The BMD is calculated by determining the reduction in radiation detected, which is related to the number of minerals available within the bone to absorb the radiation. This will give a measure of BMD in grams of hydroxyapatite/cm^2 as a proportion of an internal standard.

TABLE 3.4 The diagnosis of osteoporotic bone disease is achieved using the calculated T-score. Different degrees of bone damage are determinable

T-score	Diagnosis
Greater than −1	Normal
−1.0 → −2.5	Osteopenia
Below −2.5	Osteoporosis

● T-score: number of standard deviations the BMD deviates from the population average for healthy individuals with peak bone mass.

The WHO definition of osteoporosis is based on the T-scores (Table 3.4), as with increasing age many individuals will have normal bone density for their age and therefore a normal Z-score.

ULTRASOUND

Ultrasound is an economical and non-invasive imaging procedure used in:

- Assessment of periarticular structures, e.g. popliteal cyst or patellar tendon
- Assessment of soft tissues, e.g. a hip joint effusion in transient synovitis of the hip
- Screening, e.g. fracture risk in patients with osteoporosis, babies for DDH
- Guiding joint aspiration and injection.

Problems with definition restrict its use, but the resolution is excellent, and it is of particular use in differentiating solid from cystic, as well as defining very small structures.

CT

CT allows 3D imaging of otherwise visually problematic areas, e.g. complex intra-articular fractures, spinal canal and facet joints, as well as showing alterations in calcified anatomy. There are, however, limits to the use of CT scans due to a large radiation exposure and inadequate soft tissue visualization.

MRI

MRI gives highly detailed, multiplanar information on changes to bone and intra-articular structures such as cartilage without using ionizing radiation. Gadolinium enhancement of inflamed tissue is possible. It has a high sensitivity for change and is hence of particular use in the advanced recognition of joint disease where radiographs are of limited use. MRI is of use in:

- Spinal disease, e.g. prolapse, root or cord compression
- Osteonecrosis, e.g. Perthes' disease
- Soft tissue, bone and joint infection/tumour
- Intra-articular deformity and structural damage, e.g. meniscal and rotator cuff tears, knee ligament injuries.

BONE BIOPSY

Bone biopsy is the definitive investigation in providing the histological diagnosis for bone lesions. It is commonly performed within specialist centres, with meticulous planning and pre-biopsy imaging essential, e.g. radiographs, CT, MRI, isotope bone scan. Biopsy may be done under imaging guidance using ultrasound, CT or MRI. When a biopsy sample is collected it will be sent for histological analysis to be undertaken by an expert histopathologist, with microbiological analysis sometimes indicated, e.g. for chronic abscesses and caseating bone infections such as tuberculosis.

ARTHROSCOPY

Arthroscopy is now used in both the diagnosis and repair of soft tissue problems within the joint, commonly of the shoulder or knee. Potential complications include bleeding, damage to the joint or infection.

REGIONAL ORTHOPAEDICS AND TRAUMA

Fracture classification, general initial assessment and management, and complications are discussed in Chapter 7.

SHOULDER AND ARM

FRACTURE OF THE CLAVICLE

A clavicular fracture often occurs at the point between the middle and distal thirds, with inferior displacement of the distal fragment of the fracture due to the effect of gravity on the arm, whereas the sternomastoid muscle displaces the proximal fragment superiorly.

Clinical presentation
- Common in young males
- Direct fall onto the shoulder or FOOSH
- Shoulder and clavicular region pain and tenderness
- Visible protrusion along clavicular line, skin tenting and open fracture possible
- It is essential to assess the neurovascular status – in particular, assess brachial plexus, subclavian vessels, axillary nerve and artery status.

Investigations
- Clavicle radiograph (AP):
  — position and deformity (Figure 4.1).

Treatment
- Conservative:
  — immobilization (sling or collar and cuff) is usually sufficient
  — physiotherapy.

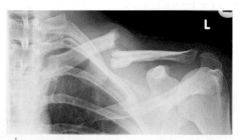

Figure 4.1 Displaced fracture of the mid-shaft of the left clavicle.

- Surgical:
    — open reduction and internal fixation (screws and plate)
    — considered for lateral fractures, open fractures, soft tissue
    (neurovascular) compromise, bilateral fractures, multiple
    trauma e.g. flail chest, and symptomatic non-unions.

Complications
- Malunion (impinged shoulder abduction) or non-union (~5%)
- Brachial plexus injury (high-energy)
- Pneumothorax injury (high-energy).

SHOULDER DISLOCATION

Injuries to the sternoclavicular and acromioclavicular (Rockwood
classification) joints are rare but when they do occur they often
involve subluxation or dislocation of the joint surface. These can
often be treated with a broad arm sling, providing there is no
neurovascular compromise and limited displacement.
Osteoarthritis is a potential complication.
  Glenohumeral joint dislocation is the commonest form of
dislocation as it is a shallow and intrinsically unstable joint. The
stability of the joint is maintained by the glenoid labrum and the
capsule, ligaments and rotator cuff muscles, which hold the
humeral head against the flat glenoid.

Anterior glenohumeral dislocation
The cause of an anterior dislocation is often traumatic (a fall
backward onto an out-stretched hand i.e. when the shoulder is
forced into abduction and external rotation) with head
displacement in the anterior–inferior direction (~95%). The forward
displacement of the humeral head often leads to injury of the
labrum and anterior capsule.

Clinical presentation
- Post acute injury, e.g. rugby player
- Intense shoulder pain with a restricted (often no) range of
  movement
- Affected fixed arm supported by opposite arm
- Gross deformity: regular lateral contour lost (more a square
  shape on presentation) with a palpable step and bulge (humeral
  head)

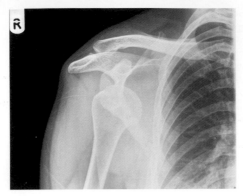

Figure 4.2 Anterior dislocation of the right shoulder joint.

- It is essential to assess the neurovascular status of the affected limb before and after reduction – in particular, assess axillary nerve (regimental badge sign and deltoid function) and artery status.

Investigations
- Shoulder radiograph (AP and axillary or 'Y' views):
  — humeral head will often be visible medially and inferiorly to the glenoid (Figure 4.2)
  — coexisting proximal humeral fracture (greater tuberosity).

Treatment
- Conservative:
  — immediate reduction with analgesia and sedation using Kochers (traction, external rotation, adduction, internal rotation), Milche's or Hippocratic method is the norm; remember a check radiograph post reduction
  — immobilization (e.g. collar and cuff)
  — physiotherapy.
- Surgical:
  — arthroscopic exploration and stabilization for young professional athletes.

Complications
- Post reduction:
  — axillary nerve damage or humeral head fracture.
- Recurrent dislocation:
  — 80% due to damage to labrum and capsule (see below).
- Rotator cuff tear (e.g. subscapularis) and stiffness:
  — elderly.

- Axillary nerve neurapraxia ('regimental patch sign'):
  — brachial plexus damage also possible.

Posterior glenohumeral dislocation

Posterior dislocations are rare and often occur following a seizure, (epileptics) or post-electrocution. This causes a direct blow to the anterior aspect of the shoulder that forces the arm into abduction and internal rotation, with head displacement in the posterior–inferior direction.

Clinical presentation
- Intense shoulder pain with no range of movement
- Arm held in internal rotation.

Investigations
- Shoulder radiograph (AP and axillary or 'Y' views):
  — AP is often normal apart from the 'light bulb sign' (Figure 4.3)
  — confirm with axillary/lateral view.
- CT or MRI if necessary.

Treatment
- Immediate reduction (often under GA) using closed (traction and external rotation) or open method
- Immobilization
- Same as anterior treatment thereafter.

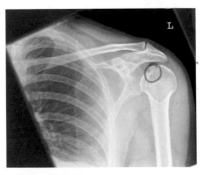

Figure 4.3 The 'light bulb sign' is clear with a rotated humeral head in the AP view. A Hill–Sachs lesion is visible on the surface of the humeral head. A CT scan will help define such a lesion.

Recurrent glenohumeral dislocation

Recurrent dislocation is often anterior and occurs due to the following processes of the original dislocation:

- Posterolateral indentation fracture of the humeral head (Hill–Sachs lesion; see Figure 4.3)
- Capsule and labrum damage at the anterior joint margin (Bankart lesion)
- Elderly with rotator cuff disease
- Atraumatic, e.g. Ehlers–Danlos syndrome.

↳ connective tissue disease: ↑motility of joints + ↑elasticity of skin.

Clinical presentation
- As before
- Positive apprehension test.

Investigations
- Shoulder radiograph (AP and axillary or 'Y' views):
  — to view dislocation as before
  — see above mentioned lesions (Figure 4.3).
- CT or MRI if necessary.

Treatment
- Conservative:
  — self-reduction sometimes possible
  — immobilization (e.g. collar and cuff)
  — physiotherapy.
- Surgical:
  — anterior capsule reconstruction for anterior dislocation (Bankart's, Putti–Platt, inferior capsular shift operations)
  — posterior dislocation requires bone and soft tissue reconstruction.

SLAP: superior labrum tear from anterior to posterior

HUMERAL FRACTURES

See Table 4.1.

ROTATOR CUFF DISEASE

A sheet of joined tendons that make up the rotator cuff covers the shoulder capsule and inserts into the greater and lesser tuberosities of the humerus. The muscles of the rotator cuff are:

- Subscapularis (internal rotation)
- Infraspinatus (external rotation)

TABLE 4.1 The subtypes, presentation and management of humeral fractures*

Subtype	Clinically	Treatment (Complications)
Proximal Humeral head Greater tuberosity Lesser tuberosity Surgical neck	Elderly, osteoporosis Fall onto shoulder/arm (direct blow) or FOOSH Assess for deformity, bruising (haemarthrosis), rotator cuff, dislocation, axillary nerve and vascular status Radiograph (Neer classification) CT may be required	Analgesia and physiotherapy Minimal displacement: immobilization Severe displacement/unstable: surgery considered, e.g. reduction and internal fixation, hemi-arthroplasty Fracture-dislocation: surgery considered (Axillary nerve/artery injury, brachial plexus injury, stiffness, dislocation, non-union, avascular necrosis of humeral head)
Shaft	Elderly, FOOSH, twisting mechanism Assess for deformity, radial nerve and vascular status Radiograph	Analgesia and physiotherapy Minimal displacement (≤20° AP): U-slab Severe displacement/unstable: surgery considered e.g. ORIF with a plate or intramedullary nail (Radial nerve injury pre- and post-op, non-union)

* AP, lateral/axial views are required for thorough assessment of the proximal humerus. Displacement is defined as a significant fragment that is angulated >45° and/or displaced >1 cm.

- Supraspinatus (abduction)
- Teres minor (external rotation and adduction).

The laxity and stability of the glenohumeral joint are determined by the stability of these muscles and the sheath of tendons associated with them. Rotator cuff disease, a degeneration of these tendons – in particular the avascular region near the insertion of the supraspinatus tendon – is commonly seen after 40 years of age, and can lead to a partial or complete tear of the tendon(s). Rotator cuff disease (that commonly involves supraspinatus) presents due to degeneration, injury or a revascularization/calcium deposition reaction:

- Rotator cuff tears as a result of trauma or chronic impingement
- Acute calcific tendinitis
- Impingement of cuff against coracoacromial arch
- Frozen shoulder (adhesive capsulitis).

Clinical presentation (Table 4.2)
- Complete tears of supraspinatus present with:
  — inability to initiate abduction but limited active abduction is possible due to scapular rotation and deltoid abduction.

Investigations
- Radiographs:
  — tears: degenerative changes
  — impingement: subacromial sclerosis
  — calcific tendinitis: calcific deposit.
- USS
- MRI or MRI-arthrography if necessary.

Treatment (Table 4.2)
- Conservative:
  — immobilization (e.g. collar and cuff) if necessary
  — physiotherapy
  — corticosteroid injection of tendon or subacromial bursa.
- Surgical:
  — arthroscopic subacromial rotator cuff decompression and debridement
  — arthroscopic or open repair, often reserved for complete tears.

TABLE 4.2 The subtypes, presentation and management of rotator cuff disease

Subtype	Clinically	Treatment
Rotator cuff impingement	Middle-aged Full range of passive movement Painful arc test positive	Physiotherapy and NSAIDs Subacromial steroid injection Subacromial decompression (recurrence)
Rotator cuff tear	Middle-aged or elderly Identify affected muscle using tests described in chapter 2 Confirm on ultrasound or MRI	Individualized
Frozen shoulder (adhesive capsulitis)	Middle-aged with IHD or DM Common post minor trauma or immobilization Limited passive movement (Loss of external rotation)	Physiotherapy and NSAIDs Distension arthrogram Arthroscopic surgical release
Calcific tendonitis	Middle-aged Full range of passive movement Severe pain Shoulder radiograph: calcific deposit	Rest and NSAIDs Subacromial steroid injection Subacromial decompression with deposit removal (recurrence)

Adapted from Surgery 24:11 (2006). Subacromial bursitis is seen as an early stage of rotator cuff tendonitis (impingement), commonly seen in younger patients. For how to assess, the muscles of the rotator cuff please see Chapter 2.

ELBOW AND FOREARM

ELBOW DISLOCATION

An elbow dislocation is commonly characterized by a posterior (most common; anterior and medial/lateral possible) displacement of the olecranon following a fall onto an outstretched hand with the elbow in flexion.   FOOSH + elbow flex

Clinical presentation
- Elbow pain and swelling with a restricted range of movement
- Gross deformity often apparent:
  — elbow triangle symmetry lost (olecranon and condyles) with olecranon prominent
  — elbow held in flexion by other arm.
- It is essential to assess the neurovascular status of the affected limb before and after reduction:
  — in particular, assess median/ulnar nerve and brachial artery status.

Investigations
- Elbow radiograph (AP and lateral):
  — position of dislocation (Figure 4.4)
  — coexisting fracture(s) not uncommon, e.g. of the radial head or coronoid process.

Treatment
- Conservative:
  — immediate reduction with analgesia and sedation; remember a check radiograph post reduction
  — immobilization (e.g. above-elbow back slab with elbow at 90°, collar and cuff)
  — physiotherapy.

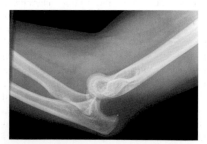

Figure 4.4 Posterior dislocation of the elbow.

- Surgical:
  — considered for fracture-dislocations with internal fixation of significant intra-articular or unstable fractures, with ligament repair sometimes needed.

Complications
- Instability:
  — persistent early instability can be treated with elbow exercises and/or a hinged external fixator.
- Stiffness, pain and/or delayed recovery of function: *calcification of muscles*
  — heterotopic ossification or myositis ossificans
  — osteoarthritis. ↳ *bony growths/calcification*
- Neurovascular injury:
  — median, radial and/or ulnar nerve neurapraxia
  — brachial artery (rare).
- Recurrent dislocation
- Post reduction:
  — neurovascular damage.

INJURIES TO THE RADIUS AND ULNA

Complex elbow fractures and fracture-dislocations
These fractures are commonly seen as a result of direct trauma (fall onto elbow). An example is the so-called terrible triad injury (posterior elbow dislocation, radial head fracture, coronoid fracture). These often require operative intervention e.g. screw/plate fixation or tension band wiring.

Fractures of the radial head
This injury is usually seen with a FOOSH. Radial neck fractures are more common in children. Radial head fractures are often difficult to see on plain radiographs (Mason classification), but haemarthrosis may cause the fat pad sign (see Figure 6.6), which, when taken in conjunction with the clinical findings (inability to fully extend the elbow, reduced range of pronation and supination), helps to make the diagnosis. It can vary widely in severity from a fine crack which is best managed with a collar and cuff followed by early movement, to a displaced and/or comminuted fracture with associated medial ligament damage and instability, which requires excision of the radial head ±prosthesis (not in children). However, some prefer open reduction and internal fixation if possible. Complications include instability, stiffness and osteoarthritis.

Fractures of the ulnar and radial shaft

These fractures are commonly seen as a result of direct trauma but are uncommon in adults. They are often compound and displaced, commonly involving both bones or one bone and one radioulnar joint. It is therefore essential that both the elbow and wrist are imaged radiologically. For example:

- Monteggia's fracture-dislocation: ulnar (proximal) fracture plus head of radius dislocation
- Galeazzi fracture-dislocation: radial (shaft) fracture plus distal ulnar dislocation.

In children, fractures tend to be greenstick with angulation so closed reduction followed by immobilization with the elbow at a right angle in a plaster cast is often successful. However, in adults open reduction and internal fixation is the preferred treatment, as it allows good alignment to optimize supination and pronation. A plaster cast is then applied. Complications include neurovascular injury (radial or posterior interosseous nerve), stiffness and decreased ROM.

Colles' fracture (distal radial fracture)

A Colles' fracture is often seen in elderly osteoporotic postmenopausal women, who have suffered a low-energy fall onto the palmar aspect of the hand (FOOSH).

Clinical presentation

- Wrist pain and swelling with a restricted range of movement
- 'Dinner-fork' wrist deformity due to shortening (radial) and angulation
- It is essential to assess the neurovascular status of the affected limb – in particular, assess median/ulnar nerve and radial artery status.

Investigations

- Wrist radiographs (AP and lateral) (Figure 4.5):
  — look for displacement, angulation, impaction and associated fracture (avulsion, intra-articular, Barton's fracture – intra-articular distal radial fracture with dislocation of the radiocarpal joint)
  — may still treat even if no fracture seen (clinical fracture).

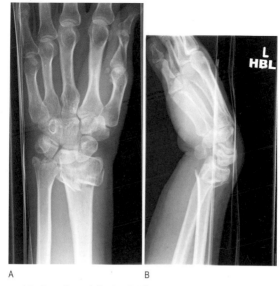

A   B

Figure 4.5 Comminuted distal radial fracture (within 2.5 cm of wrist joint) with dorsal and radial displacement, impaction and an associated avulsion fracture of the ulnar styloid. (**A**) AP; (**B**) lateral.

Treatment
- Conservative:
  — immediate reduction using a regional block (e.g. Bier's) if displaced; remember a check radiograph post reduction (often repeated at 1 week)
  — immobilization (e.g. Colles' forearm dorsal plaster slab)
  — physiotherapy.
- Surgical:
  — considered if closed reduction and immobilization have not worked (instability) or if complicated fractures (intra-articular, comminuted, open, concomitant carpal injury)
  — percutaneous K-wire fixation or external fixation for unstable fractures
  — open reduction and fixation for intra-articular fractures
  — bone grafting and internal fixation for radial collapse.

Complications
- Post reduction:
  — neurovascular damage.

- Postoperative:
  — osteomyelitis
  — flexor pollicis longus tendon rupture.
- Stiffness, pain and deformity:
  — hand oedema
  — reflex sympathetic dystrophy (Sudeck's atrophy)
  — malunion often with associated angulation (corrected by osteotomy).
- Neurovascular and soft tissue injury:
  — median (acute carpal tunnel syndrome) and/or ulnar nerve neuropraxia
  — radial and/or ulnar artery (rare)
  — extensor pollicis longus tendon rupture (delayed complication)
  — wrist ligament strain.

Smith's fracture

A Smith's fracture is characterized by a transverse extra-articular distal radial fracture near the radiocarpal joint, with *volar angulation and displacement of the distal portion. Clinical presentation* is common after a fall onto the dorsal aspect of the hand. Wrist pain and swelling with a restricted range of movement are seen. *Treatment* is with splint immobilization, after reduction if displaced. Internal fixation with a plate e.g. a buttress plate, is often necessary due to instability.

TENNIS ELBOW

Tennis elbow, or lateral epicondylitis, is the chronic inflammation, degeneration and rupture of aponeurotic fibres of the common extensor tendon where it originates from the lateral supracondylar ridge of the humerus. It is commonly caused by minor trauma or repetitive strain occurring when the extensors of the arm are contracted, accompanied by sharp flexion of the wrist, e.g. a backhand stroke in tennis.

Clinical presentation
- Middle-aged
- Pain at the lateral condyle, tender to touch
- Reproducible pain if patient's wrist is extended against resistance
- Normal flexion and extension of the elbow.

Treatment
- Conservative:
  - analgesia e.g. NSAIDs
  - physiotherapy
  - corticosteroid injection.
- Surgical:
  - rarely indicated
  - common extensor origin stripping and release.

GOLFER'S ELBOW

Golfer's elbow, or medial epicondylitis, is the chronic inflammation, degeneration and rupture of aponeurotic fibres of the common flexor tendon where it originates from the medial supracondylar ridge of the humerus. Pain is commonly caused by strain occurring with hyperextension of the wrist and fingers, e.g. a golfer striking the ground, not the ball. It is less common than tennis elbow.

Clinical presentation
- Pain at the medial condyle, tender to touch
- Tenderness area less precise than with tennis elbow
- Normal flexion and extension of the elbow
- Reproducible pain on resisted wrist flexion.

Treatment
- Conservative:
  - analgesia e.g. NSAIDs
  - - physiotherapy
  - corticosteroid injection.
- Surgical:
  - rarely indicated
  - common flexor origin stripping and release.

WRIST AND HAND

SCAPHOID FRACTURE

A scaphoid fracture is common after a fall onto the hand with a dorsiflexed wrist FOOSH, accounting for three-quarters of all carpal bone fractures. It is not commonly seen in the extremes of age, but there is a male predominance.

Clinical presentation
- Wrist pain and swelling with sometimes a restricted range of movement
- Tenderness notable on gripping and wrist extension
- Tender and full anatomical snuffbox, the borders of which are:
  — proximal = radial styloid
  — posterior/medial = extensor pollicis longus tendon
  — anterior/lateral = extensor pollicis brevis and APL tendon
  — distal = mid-point of the thumb metacarpal.
- Assess the neurovascular status of the affected hand – in particular, assess radial artery status.

Investigations
- Scaphoid view radiographs (AP, lateral and two oblique):
  — fracture, most commonly seen at waist (Figure 4.6)
  — ligament damage along with displacement
  — repeat radiograph at 2 weeks if fracture not seen and still treat if clinical fracture.

Treatment
- Conservative:
  — immobilization (e.g. scaphoid/thumb-spica cast even if clinical only and review at 2 weeks)
  — physiotherapy.

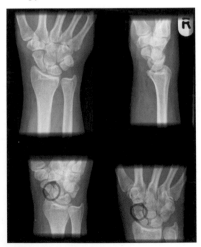

Figure 4.6 Fracture through the waist of the scaphoid (scaphoid radiograph views). Less common are proximal pole fractures that give the highest risk of avascular necrosis. Distal scaphoid fractures are rare.

- Surgical:
  — considered if there is instability, displacement, angulation, or concomitant carpal dislocation
  — percutaneous K-wire fixation
  — open reduction and percutaneous compression screw fixation
  — bone grafting and internal fixation for delayed or non-union.

Complications
- Stiffness and pain
- Neurovascular and soft tissue injury:
  — trans-scaphoid perilunate dislocation.
- Proximal bone avascular necrosis (30%):
  — blood supply occurs from the distal to proximal pole
  — secondary OA.
- Non-union:
  — scaphoid extends from the proximal to the distal row of carpal bones
  — secondary OA.

CARPAL DISLOCATION

Carpal dislocations do occur and should not be missed; the most frequent is a lunate dislocation (dislocation of the radiolunate joint). *Clinical presentation* is common after a fall onto an outstretched hand. Wrist pain, swelling and deformity can be seen with a restricted range of movement. Assessment of neurovascular status is essential, in particular the median nerve. AP and lateral wrist radiographs are essential. *Treatment* is with immobilization, after reduction (closed or open with K-wire fixation) if displaced (often anteriorly). Be aware of avascular necrosis and OA of the lunate in particular. Dislocation of the lunate (remains aligned with radius) from the capitate is known as a perilunate dislocation.

FOOSH

BENNETT'S FRACTURE-SUBLUXATION

Bennett's fracture-subluxation is a thumb metacarpal base intra-articular fracture with proximal and radial displacement of the major fragment of the metacarpal.

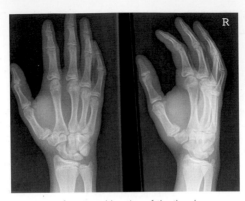

Figure 4.7 Bennett's fracture-subluxation of the thumb.

proximal + radial displacement.

Clinical presentation
- Thumb base pain and swelling
- Range of movement at the thumb CMCJ is reduced with instability often apparent
- Assess neurovascular status of the affected thumb.

Investigations
- Thumb radiographs (AP, lateral and oblique):
  — fracture and instability (Figure 4.7)
  — repeat radiograph at 2 weeks if fracture not seen (scaphoid views to exclude fracture).

Treatment
- Conservative:
  — closed reduction with analgesia/ring block
  — immobilization (e.g. Bennett's cast)
  — physiotherapy.
- Surgical:
  — often considered due to instability or if malpositioned
  — open reduction and screw or percutaneous wire fixation.

Complications
- Pain and stiffness:
  — long-term risk of secondary OA if degree of injury to CMCJ is severe.

THUMB COLLATERAL LIGAMENT INJURY (GAMEKEEPER'S THUMB)

Now more commonly known as skier's thumb, this is a rupture of the ulnar collateral ligament of the thumb. *Clinical presentation* is common after a fall (abduction force) onto an extended thumb. The patient will have a painful and swollen thumb with a restricted range of movement. Tenderness will be noted over the ulnar aspect of the thumb MCPJ, but attempt to assess both collateral ligaments, perhaps after local anaesthetic injection. AP and lateral/stress view radiographs of the thumb are recommended to exclude a fracture. *Treatment* is immobilization with a thumb spica followed by physiotherapy if only a partial rupture is suspected. A complete rupture and/or a fracture often requires operative repair.

METACARPAL FRACTURES

Metacarpal fractures account for 30–50% of all hand fractures and can be differentiated into: (1) thumb metacarpal head, shaft and base fractures; and (2) finger metacarpal head, neck, shaft and base fractures. Fractures of the 5th metacarpal account for 60% of these fractures. The variety of injury mechanisms leading to fracture ranges from axial loading due to falls to direct dorsal blows to the hand (Boxer's fracture). Associated subsequent deformities of the hand following fracture include shortening, angulation and malrotation, along with soft tissue injury and swelling.

↳ #metacarpal neck,
commonly 5th (or 4th)

Clinical presentation
- Metacarpal pain and swelling
- Deformity if displaced fracture:
  — flattened knuckle or protrusion on dorsal aspect of the hand.
- Bite marks over 5th knuckle:
  — human post punch, prone to aerobic and/or anaerobic infection.

Investigations
- Hand radiograph (AP, lateral and oblique):
  — fracture and displacement (Figure 4.8).

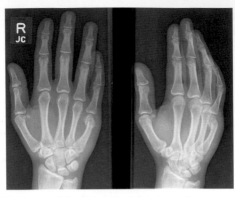

Figure 4.8 Fracture of the neck of the 5th metacarpal.

↳ " Boxer's # "

Treatment
● Conservative:
  — a vast number of metacarpal fractures are closed injuries, adequately treated by immobilization, with or without closed reduction as necessary
  — immobilization (e.g. tubigrip, neighbour strapping, plaster as required)
  — physiotherapy.
● Surgical:
  — considered if there is significant displacement/deformity and/or comminution
  — mandatory exploration washout joint is penetrated
  — percutaneous pin fixation is the bridge between closed and open reduction
  — ORIF is considered for unstable, open, multiple, malaligned or simply irreducible fracture patterns.

Complications
● Postoperative infection
● Stiffness and pain:
  — OA
  — disability of the hand.
● Non-union
● Malunion:
  — rotational deformity leading to disability of the hand. mandatory exploration washout.

INJURY TO THE PHALANGES

Fractures of the phalanges

Fractures and/or dislocations to the phalanges often follow direct trauma. Crush fractures of the distal phalanges are not uncommon and may be compound. *Clinical presentation* is often with pain, swelling and possibly deformity over the affected area. Assess the soft tissues of the affected finger, in particular the digital artery and nerve, as well as the long extensor and flexor tendons of the finger. AP and lateral views of individual fingers are needed. *Treatment* is with reduction if necessary, splint immobilization neighbour strapping and early physiotherapy. Nailbed deformities should be treated as appropriate, e.g. trephining a subungual haematoma, and antibiotics and/or tetanus are important to consider in compound fractures of the distal phalanx. Fixation with K-wires is indicated if there is fracture instability.

Mallet finger

Mallet finger is caused by a blow to an actively extended finger, leading to extensor tendon rupture ± avulsion from the base of the distal phalanx. (A boutonnière deformity is the presentation when the central slip of extensor tendon ruptures.) *Clinical presentation* is often of a finger which is seen flexed at the DIPJ, with no extension possible (passive extension is possible). History of trauma, e.g. catching a ball, is common. AP and lateral views of the affected finger are needed. *Treatment* is with splint immobilization (mallet splint) of the DIPJ in hyperextension. Fixation and/or arthrodesis are indicated if there is significant displaced fracture or if there is a severe deformity post splintage.

[handwritten annotation: DIPJ hyperext. PIPJ flex.]

CARPAL TUNNEL SYNDROME

Carpal tunnel syndrome is the compression and subsequent ischaemia of the median nerve as it enters the hand under the flexor retinaculum (transverse carpal ligament) of the carpal tunnel. Middle-aged women (8 : 1) are most commonly affected.

Risk factors

- Fluid retention: pregnancy, combined oral contraceptive pill
- Musculoskeletal: RA or OA
- Endocrine: diabetes mellitus, obesity, hypothyroidism, myxoedema, acromegaly, congestive cardiac failure
- Trauma: distal radius or carpal bone fracture, e.g. lunate.

Clinical presentation (due to median nerve compression)

- Pain and paraesthesia of the median distribution (thumb, index, middle and the radial half of the ring fingers), more marked at night; pain often relieved by shaking hand
- Lateral aspect of palm spared as superficial palmar branch is given off proximal to flexor retinaculum
- Thenar muscle wasting (in advanced cases).

Investigations

- Phalen's test (hyperflexed wrist for 2 mins will reproduce symptoms)
- Tinel's test (tapping in region of nerve on anterior wrist crease) is less sensitive
- Nerve conduction study.

Treatment

- Conservative:
  - rest
  - immobilization (extension wrist splints)
  - corticosteroid injection (maximum of three attempts advised).
- Surgical:
  - surgery entails carpal tunnel decompression by flexor retinaculum division.

DUPUYTREN'S CONTRACTURE

Dupuytren's contracture, first described in 1831 by a Parisian surgeon, is a progressive, painless fibrotic thickening of the palmar and digital fascia (aponeurosis), leading to nodular hypertrophy and contracture of the fascia. The clinical picture is a hand contracture that commences at the base of the ring and little finger, leading to skin puckering and tethering, with fixed flexion deformity of these fingers. It is more common in men (10 : 1).

Risk factors

- Alcoholism and liver disease
- Smoking
- Epilepsy/antiepileptic drugs, e.g. phenytoin therapy
- Diabetes mellitus
- AIDS/HIV
- Family history (autosomal dominant pattern).

Clinical presentation

- Bilateral and symmetrical
- Pain uncommon

- Puckered, nodular thickening of the palm
- Contracture of MCP and PIP joints of the ring and little fingers
- Hueston tabletop test positive, i.e. cannot place hand flat and open on table.

Treatment
- Conservative:
  — none effective
  — in trial is non-invasive enzyme fasciotomy.
- Surgical:
  — considered if patient has palmar infection or is disabled with deformity, e.g. cannot place palm flat on a table
  — fasciotomy or partial fasciectomy of the palmar fascia
  — skin grafting may be needed
  — postoperative splinting and physiotherapy.

Complications
- Recurrence common
- Postoperative:
  — infection
  — neurovascular injury
  — swelling due to oedema, haematoma.
- Stiffness and pain:
  — reflex sympathetic dystrophy (Sudeck's atrophy)
  — loss of function.

↳ bone pain, swelling + localited OP.

DE QUERVAIN'S TENOSYNOVITIS

De Quervain's tenosynovitis, first described in 1895 by a Swiss surgeon, is an inflammation and stenosis of the tendon sheaths of abductor pollicis longus and extensor pollicis brevis. Inflammation and pain commonly occur secondary to a repetitive movement. It is also associated with inflammatory arthritis. It is commonly seen in middle-aged women.

Clinical presentation
- Wrist and thumb pain on use, but often with full range of movement
- Pain at site of inflammation, as the tendons pass between the radial styloid and the overlying extensor retinaculum
- Finkelstein's test reproduces the pain:
  — flexion of the thumb across the palm
  — encompass with fist
  — then ulnar deviation of the wrist.

Treatment
- Conservative:
  — rest and immobilization
  — corticosteroid injection.
- Surgical:
  — division and release of the tendon sheath.

Complications
- Postoperative: radial nerve neurapraxia
- Radial-carpal instability
- Recurrence.

PELVIS, HIP AND KNEE

PELVIC AND ACETABULAR FRACTURES

Fractures to the pelvic ring or acetabulum commonly occur following RTAs or when elderly people fall (public rami fractures). Severe unstable fractures are associated with considerable blood loss, particularly when there is injury to the pubic symphysis and/ or posterior osseous–ligamentous complex (open pelvic ring). The Young and Burgess classification is often used for pelvic fractures (lateral compression, AP compression, vertical shear, combined). Displacement of the pelvis can lead to urogenital injury.

Clinical presentation
- Pain and bruising in the pelvic region
- Pelvic instability (check may be contraindicated)
- Flank, perianal and urogenital swelling, bruising and bleeding
- Per rectum examination may reveal a high-riding prostate
- It is essential to assess the distal neurology – in particular, assess the sciatic and inferior/superior gluteal nerves.

Investigations
- Pelvic radiograph (AP, inlet/outlet views and oblique views for the acetabulum)
- CT of the pelvis:
  — often definitive
  — urogenital assessment possible.

Treatment
- ATLS assessment and resuscitation
- Pelvic stabilization using as external fixator (prevents clot disruption and thus helps to control haemorrhage)

— Radiological embolization may be required
- Conservative:
  — pelvic stabilization with an external fixator
  — physiotherapy.
- Surgical:
  — definitive fixation individualized, with operative intervention often indicated for unstable pelvic fractures and for intra-articular acetabular disruption.

Complications
- Malunion and OA (acetabular fractures)
- Urogenital and rectal injury and dysfunction
- Neurovascular injury; sciatic nerve neurapraxia

HIP DISLOCATION

Hip dislocation is commonly characterized by a posterior displacement of the femoral head following a blow to the thigh with the hip in flexion and adduction, e.g. a direct blow to the knee on a dashboard.

Clinical presentation
- Hip pain and swelling with a restricted range of movement.
- Gross deformity often apparent:
  — loss of normal skin crease
  — posterior: hip is flexed, adducted, shortened and internally rotated
  — anterior: hip is flexed, abducted and externally rotated.
- It is essential to assess the neurovascular status of the affected limb before and after reduction
  — in particular, assess the sciatic nerve.

Investigations
- Hip, femur and knee radiographs (AP and lateral):
  — position of dislocation (Thompson–Epstein classification)
  — coexisting injury, e.g. acetabular fracture, femoral head fracture, femoral shaft fracture, PCL injury of the knee.

Treatment
- Conservative:
  — immediate reduction under GA; remember a check radiograph (or CT scan) post reduction

— immobilization (rest) and traction
— physiotherapy.
● Surgical:
— considered for fracture-dislocations, e.g. displaced fracture of acetabulum.

Complications
● Recurrence
● Avascular necrosis: secondary OA
● Neurovascular injury: sciatic nerve neurapraxia.

PROXIMAL FEMORAL FRACTURES

Fractures of the femoral neck are often caused by a blow to the greater trochanter and occur following severe trauma (RTA) in the young, and minor trauma (fall) in the elderly (chiefly postmenopausal osteoporotic women). ~30% patients die within 12 months of fracture. Garden's classification of hip fractures is shown in Figure 4.9.

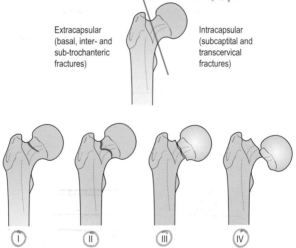

Figure 4.9 Intracapsular fractures are linked with avascular necrosis, which can be explained with knowledge of the femoral neck vasculature. The closer the fracture is to the head, the more likely the retinacular vessels will be disrupted. Garden's classification: I, impacted incomplete fracture; II, non-displaced complete fracture; III, partially displaced complete fracture; IV, fully displaced complete fracture. Displaced fractures are associated with an increased risk of complications and avascular necrosis.

The blood supply to the femoral head makes it vulnerable to developing avascular necrosis. The primary vasculatures (the nutrient, retinacular and medullary vessels) are damaged severely if there is an intracapsular fracture of the neck, leaving the ligamentum teres as the single source. This provides an inadequate vascular (nutrient) supply, leading to ischaemic necrosis and collapse of the femoral head.

Extracapsular hip fractures commonly occur between the greater and lesser trochanters, i.e. intertrochanteric fractures. Less common are subtrochanteric fractures.

Clinical presentation
- History of trauma, e.g. fall or RTA
- Hip pain with little or no weight bearing or movements possible
- Displaced fractures cause external rotation and shortening of the leg.

Investigations
- Hip and pelvic radiographs (AP and lateral) (Figure 4.10):
  — Shenton's line (really a parabolic curve) runs along the upper border of the obturator foramen and the inferior border of the femoral neck; an alteration in this line will identify any possible fracture and displacement of the hip.

Treatment
- ATLS assessment and resuscitation
- DVT prophylaxis
- If surgery contraindicated – analgesia, traction, rest and chest physio
- Surgery (Figure 4.11)

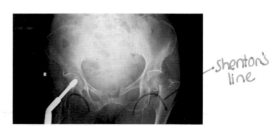

Shenton's line

Figure 4.10 An intracapsular fracture of the left neck of femur. There is a DHS in place for an old extra-capsular fracture on the right side.

↳ dynamic hip screw

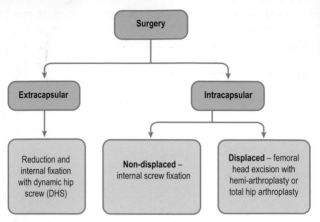

Figure 4.11 Surgical options for proximal femoral fractures. Younger patients with a displaced intracapsular fracture maybe suitable for early. reduction and intenal fixation with cannulated screws. Early mobilization postoperatively.

Complications
- Peri-operative (see Chapter 7)
  — DVT/PE, pneumonia ARF, MI, CVA
  — Post hemi-arthoplasty complications (see p 140)
  — Death (30% within 1 year)
- Non-union and malunion leading to secondary OA
- Femoral head avascular necrosis:
  — secondary OA.

FEMORAL SHAFT FRACTURE

Fractures of the femoral shaft commonly occur following high-velocity RTAs, e.g. as part of major trauma. They are associated with considerable blood loss. *Clinical presentation* is often with pain, deformity and bruising in the thigh region. It is essential to assess the soft tissues of the affected leg, in particular assess the sciatic nerve and peripheral circulation. A femoral radiograph (AP and lateral) is required. *Treatment* is with resuscitation first and fracture splinting, e.g. Thomas splint. Surgery (intramedullary nail) is often indicated. *Complications* include malunion, deformity, infection, VTE, fat embolism and stiffness.

KNEE LIGAMENT INJURY

See Table 4.3.

TABLE 4.3 The aetiology, presentation and management of knee ligament injuries*

Ligament and aetiology	Clinically	Treatment (Complications)
ACL More common in males Incidence 1 in 3000/year Common sports injury Valgus twisting, hyperextension, foot rig'd to ground, knee flexed Associated ligament and menisci injury	History of trauma Effusion and pain Decreased ROM Positive anterior draw test MRI or arthroscopy	Rest and analgesia Physiotherapy Immobilization if needed Ligament reconstruction _hamstring tendon_ Repair meniscal tear (Chronic instability, OA)
PCL Uncommon Common following RTAs (knee flexed, tibia forced posteriorly) Other ligament injury very common	History of trauma Inability to weight bear, knee gives way Positive posterior draw test MRI or arthroscopy	Rest and analgesia Physiotherapy Immobilization if needed Surgery for athletes (OA)
MCL Most common Associated ACL or medial meniscal injury Lateral blow is common (valgus stress)	History of trauma Effusion uncommon Tenderness Valgus testing positive (Grade 1–3) MRI or arthroscopy to confirm	Rest and analgesia Physiotherapy Immobilization if needed Surgery if unstable or chronic
LCL Uncommon Medial blow is common ~~(valgus stress)~~ _varus stress_ Associated with ACL and PCL injury Associated with biceps femoris tendon, fascia lata and common peroneal nerve injury	Instability less common LCL not easily found Varus testing positive (Grade 1–3) MRI or arthroscopy to confirm	Rest and analgesia Physiotherapy Immobilization if needed Surgery rarely needed

* Ligament injuries often follow a twisting injury or a direct blow to the medial or lateral aspect of the knee. The pain will often extend beyond the joint line to the ligament insertions. Rapidly developing effusions are often associated with ligament injuries as they are highly vascular (haemarthrosis). Ligament strain is associated with a stable joint and a more modest effusion. Meniscal injuries often present with a slower developing effusion also.

MENISCAL INJURY

Damage to these fibrocartilaginous load-bearing structures can be acute (normal menisci, damage due to twisting, common following sports injury) or chronic (abnormal menisci, damage after little trauma, common in the elderly). A cruciate ligament tear predisposes to meniscal injury. The medial meniscus is more commonly affected than the lateral due to its decreased mobility in relation to the capsule. However, a lateral meniscal injury will more likely lead to degenerative changes due to the convex shape of the lateral tibial plateau. Men are more frequently affected. Six common types of meniscal tear occur:

1. Radial
2. Bucket-handle
3. Flap
4. Horizontal cleavage (common in degenerated menisci)
5. Vertical
6. Degenerative.

*[handwritten: acute = med. meniscus
chronic = lat. menisus (degenerative)]*

The position of the tear is of clinical relevance in terms of ability to heal due to varying vascular supply, i.e. the more peripheral the tear the greater the chance of repair due to an increased vascular supply. *Clinical presentation* is common in sports, particularly during contact. Joint line pain and tenderness, a locked knee, swelling (effusion) or a meniscal cyst (one-way valve synovial leak) may be seen. The diagnosis is clinically apparent (McMurray's or Apley's positive) in up to 70%, but MRI and arthroscopy can be used to confirm the diagnosis. Associated ligament injury may be present. *Treatment* is initially with RICE, analgesia and physiotherapy. Surgery (arthroscopy) involves either repair or partial meniscectomy. *Complications* of surgery include infection (<1%) and OA in large meniscectomies.

EXTENSOR MECHANISM INJURY

This injury is due either to fracture of the patella (transverse), or to rupture of the patellar tendon (ligamentum patellae) or quadriceps muscle/tendon. Fracture of the patella may present similarly. *Clinical presentation* is often with knee pain, swelling, tenderness and a gap at the point of rupture. Inability to straight leg raise is common. A knee radiograph (AP and lateral) will show if the patella is high (patella tendon rupture) or low (quadriceps tear). *Treatment* is with immobilization ± operative repair for tendon rupture or avulsion (e.g. from the tibial tubercle).

INJURIES TO THE PATELLA

Fractures of the patella

Brisk contraction of the quadriceps against resistance can lead to an avulsion or transverse fracture. Direct trauma from the dashboard in an RTA or from assault with a weapon may give rise to a comminuted (stellate) fracture and/or a haemarthrosis. Fractures that do not affect the extensor mechanism and that are not comminuted or displaced can be managed in a plaster cast. Transverse fractures undergo ORIF with tension-band wiring if displaced. If the extensor mechanism is compromised, surgical repair is indicated. Patellectomy may be required. In the long term, OA of the patellofemoral compartment may develop. NB: A normal variant on X-ray is a congenital bi- or tripartite patella. This can be mistaken for a fracture but often occurs bilaterally.

Dislocation of the patella

Dislocation of the patella, and subsequent rupture of the medial patello–femoral ligament, is seen when athletes 'side-step'. It is also seen commonly in teenage girls who get recurrent dislocations, either spontaneously or with minimal trauma. In the acute setting, lateral displacement of the patella is reduced by medial pressure and knee extension under analgesia/sedation. A knee radiograph is needed to exclude an osteochondral fracture. After an initial period of rest in a plaster cast, physiotherapy to strengthen the quadriceps is required. There are several anatomical variants which predispose to recurrent dislocation (seen after 15–20% of patellar dislocations): ligament laxity, flattening of the lateral epicondyle, genu valgum and a small high-riding patella. If intensive physiotherapy to strengthen vastus medialis is not successful, surgery may be required.

INJURIES TO THE TIBIA

Fractures of the tibial plateau

This injury is often due to a direct compression i.e. femoral condyle impacting into the tibial plateau. Damage to either (lateral more common than medial) or both of the tibial condyles is often caused by compression from the opposite femoral condyle. *Clinical presentation* is with knee pain, swelling (haemarthrosis) and deformity (valgus or varus). Associated ligament injury may be apparent on stress testing. A knee radiograph will show the extent of the fracture (Schatzker's classification). CT may be required. *Treatment* is dependent on the degree of displacement and the extent of fracture(s). It can vary widely from brief immobilization and early physiotherapy, to ORIF, ligament repair or even total knee arthroplasty. *Complications* include deformity, compartment syndrome, neurovascular injury (common peroneal nerve leading to foot drop) and OA (meniscal injury).

Fractures of the tibial shaft

This fracture is often due to a large direct or indirect injury, e.g. RTA. Open fractures are common. A fibula fracture can also occur. *Treatment* is dependent on the type and stability of the fracture(s). Some stable fractures can undergo immediate reduction under GA (check radiograph post reduction), followed by immobilization and physiotherapy. Unstable or open fractures require surgery, e.g. tibial nail, external fixator, plate. *Complications* include infection, soft tissue neurovascular injury (popliteal artery, common peroneal nerve in a proximal fibular fracture), deformity, compartment syndrome, reflex sympathetic dystrophy and disunion (in particular non-union).

ANKLE AND FOOT

ANKLE AND FOOT FRACTURES

See Table 4.4.

ANKLE LIGAMENT STRAIN

Strains are characterized by damage to the anterior talofibular and calcaneofibular ligaments due to talus inversion during trauma. Lateral sprains are more common. *Clinical presentation* is common in sports, particularly rugby. Ankle pain, swelling and tenderness over the LCLs are common. Radiographs (Ottawa Ankle Rules) are only carried out if the patient cannot weight

TABLE 4.4 The subtypes, presentation and management of ankle and foot fractures*

Subtype	Clinically	Treatment* (Complications)
Ankle	Indirect injury, e.g. inversion injury of ankle Associated dislocation and ligament injury Complicated by medial ligament injury and talar shift	(Pain, Sudeck's atrophy, OA)
Weber A	Horizontal avulsion fibular fracture below syndesmosis	Immobilize in plaster
Weber B	Spiral fibular fracture at syndesmosis, possible ligament damage	Immobilize in plaster if stable
Weber C	Fracture above syndesmosis, definite ligament damage	ORIF considered for notable displacement or instability
Talus	Forced dorsiflexion High-energy trauma, e.g. RTA, fall from height Low-energy trauma, e.g. ankle sprain leading to avulsion	Immobilize in below-knee plaster ORIF for notable displacement (Avascular necrosis)
Calcaneum	Fall onto heel, bilateral not uncommon High-energy trauma, e.g. fall from height Associated with spine, pelvis and tibial plateau injury	RICE ORIF considered for notable displacement or instability Bone grafts if necessary (Deformity, OA compartment syndrome, neurovascular injury)
Metatarsal 5th Base	Inversion injury: avulsion (peroneus brevis) Direct injury: complete	Immobilize in below-knee plaster ORIF considered for notable displacement or instability
Other	Shaft, stress, neck	Treat as above

* The Ottawa Ankle Rules provide indications of when to radiograph the ankle. Always assess proximally, particularly for a proximal fibula fracture. Bi-malleolar fractures, tri-malleolar fractures, displacement (e.g. talar shift) and significant fibular injury indicate an unstable ankle injury that will likely require ORIF. If reduction and stability can be achieved in a Weber C fracture, ORIF maybe avoided.

(margin note) ability to weight bare, pain (malleoli, foot bones), >55yrs, inability to flex 90°, pain @ fibula head* or patella**

**(margin note) (knee)

bear or if there is bony tenderness, which may imply fracture/
avulsion (Weber fractures). *Treatment* is initially with RICE,
analgesia, immobilization and physiotherapy. Surgery –
reconstruction or arthroscopy – is rarely required. *Complications*:
joint instability can lead to recurrent sprains.

HALLUX VALGUS

Hallux valgus is characterized by severe lateral angulation and
rotation of the hallux, with medial deviation of the metatarsal
(metatarsus primus varus). Although primarily determined
genetically (e.g. wide forefoot, varus big toe metatarsal), pain is
exacerbated in people who chronically wear tight shoes or those
with RA. A medial bunion (metatarsal head and bursa
hypertrophy) is common. *Clinical presentation* is common in
women in their 5th, 6th and 7th decade. Bilateral deformity is
common, with pain often due to 1st MTP joint OA, tight shoes or
metatarsalgia (pain across the metatarsal heads). *Treatment* is
primarily shoe changes, e.g. wide shoes with soft uppers. Orthotic
moulded insoles can be helpful. Surgery entails first metatarsal
osteotomy (e.g. Chevron osteotomy), soft tissue realignment,
bunion excision or even joint arthrodesis. Complications include
OA, exostosis and 2nd MTPJ dislocation.

ACHILLES TENDON RUPTURE

A partial or full rupture of the Achilles tendon may occur.
Clinical presentation is often related to sports, but should be
suspected in anyone who presents with a sudden onset of pain in
the posterior aspect of their ankle and the inability to weight bear
(partially or at all). Simmons test is used to confirm rupture
(see Chapter 2). An ankle radiograph is indicated if there is a
suspected fracture of the ankle joint. A USS of the calf will
exclude a gastrocnemius muscle tear (pain often higher in mid-
calf). *Treatment* is with immobilization in equinus using a below-
knee plaster. Surgical repair of the tendon may be necessary.

Simmons → calf.squeeze + NO plantar flex.

PLANTAR FASCIITIS

Plantar fasciitis is a self-limiting inflammation of the plantar
fascia, which is often seen in middle-aged obese women. There is
an association with Reiter's disease (reactive arthritis). *Clinical*

Glasgow coma scale			
	Score		Score
Eye opening (E)		**Verbal response (V)**	
Spontaneous	4	Orientated	5
To speech	3	Confused conversation	4
To pain	2	Inappropriate words	3
No response	1	Incomprehensible sounds	2
		No response	1
Motor response (M)			
Obeys	6		
Localizes	5		
Withdraws (Normal flexion)	4		
Abnormal flexion	3		
Extension	2		
No response	1		
Glasgow Coma Scale = $E + M + V$			
(GCS minimum = 3, maximum = 15, coma ≤ 8)			

Figure 4.12 Glasgow Coma Scale.

presentation is with heel pain, worse in the morning (after rest).
Tenderness over the insertion of the plantar fascia on the
calcaneus (anteromedial aspect of the heel) is seen. *Treatment* is
with analgesia, insoles, physiotherapy, night immobilization and
local corticosteroid/anaesthetic injections.

HEAD, NECK AND SPINE

HEAD INJURIES

Head injuries are a common presentation to A&E departments
throughout the UK. Initially, if admission is necessary, these
patients will be under the care of either the general or orthopaedic
surgeons depending on the hospital to which they are admitted.
Alcohol and assault are common coexisting factors with these
patients, but it is important to remember that alcohol is not a
valid reason for an alternating conscious level. The Glasgow
Coma Score (GCS) is essential in the assessment and classification
of these patients (Figure 4.12).

Initial assessment

Important aspects of the history are:

- Mode of injury, e.g. weapon used, blunt or penetrating injury
- Neurological symptoms, e.g. severe headache, persistent nausea and vomiting, seizure activity, amnesia, loss of consciousness
- Co-morbidities, e.g. alcohol excess, previous head injuries
- Current medications, in particular anticoagulation, e.g. aspirin, clopidogrel or warfarin.

Examination should include:

- Airway, breathing, circulation (ABC)
- Disability: general and neurological observations (GCS and pupils)
- Exposure: inspection for any external signs of trauma throughout the body
- Neurological exam to exclude any focal neurology and evidence of a skull fracture, e.g. Battle's sign (retroauricular ecchymosis) or raccoon's eyes (periorbital ecchymosis) in a basal skull fracture, CSF leak, depressions
- A full general examination.

→ subcutaneous purpura aka bruise

Management (refer to local guidelines)

- As before, ATLS guidelines should be followed initially, with particular importance placed on ABC and clearing the C-spine when neck injuries are suspected:
  — ensure adequate cerebral perfusion and reduce intracranial pressure when elevated (normotonic i.v. fluids, hyperventilation, mannitol)
  — intubation method and nasogastric tube placement must be cautioned in those with a suspected basal skull fracture.
- Investigations should include:
  — alcohol reading and blood sugar
  — blood tests (e.g. sodium and glucose levels) and ECG where indicated
  — imaging (Figure 4.13).
- Admission should be considered in patients with:
  — a GCS score that is less than 15 or fluctuating
  — positive neurology, i.e. patients with persisting neurological symptoms (headache, nausea/vomiting, amnesia, irritability), seizure activity, focal neurology on examination
  — abnormal imaging

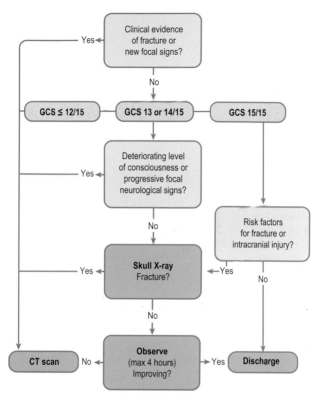

Figure 4.13 Indication for imaging during the early management of head injury. This flow chart is taken from SIGN Guideline 46: Early Management of Head Injury (currently under review), and gives advice on when a skull radiograph and/or CT head scan are required. A linear skull vault fracture increases the risk of an intracranial bleed by almost 400-fold. It should be noted that other guidelines recommend a CT head as the first choice of imaging in head injuries, and it is therefore important to refer to your locally agreed protocols and guidelines for head injury assessment and management.

aka. basal skull #

— inadequate social support or supervision
— a risk of developing an intracranial bleed, e.g. patients on warfarin.
● Regular neurological observations:
— those with persisting or worsening neurology should be considered for CT scanning.

- Drugs:
  — analgesia
  — control bleeding and complete closure of open wounds
  — avoid sedating drugs, e.g. diazepam for alcohol withdrawal
  — tetanus and prophylactic antibiotics should be considered in open injuries.
- Consider referral to neurosurgeons, e.g. intracranial lesion (diffuse brain injury, extradural/subdural/intracerebral haematomas) on imaging, deteriorating or low GCS, worsening neurology.

SPINAL FRACTURES

See Table 4.5.

NECK PAIN

Neck pain is commonly seen in the elderly, but does not have the same magnitude of effect on young people as back pain. It is not commonly associated with significant spinal pathology, but may cause devastating quadriplegia if the cervical cord is compromised.

Causes
- Mechanical neck pain
- Acute neck sprain, i.e. whiplash
- Inflammation, e.g. RA
- Bone mineral disease, e.g. osteoporosis
- Cervical disc prolapse
- Metastases
- Referred pain, e.g. diaphragm.

Clinical presentation
- Acute asymmetrical decreased ROM of neck
- History of trauma or persistent uncomfortable posture
- Assess for direct spinal tenderness
- Pain from the neck may radiate to:
  — head: temple, occiput or face
  — upper limb: scapula, shoulder or upper arm.
- Radicular pain and neurological symptoms from C6 or, less commonly, C7 or C8 compression.

TABLE 4.5 The subtypes, presentation and management of spinal fractures*

Subtype	Clinically
Cervical	Types of injury: crush, burst, wedge fractures, facet joint dislocations
	Due to direct or indirect trauma; hyperflexion, extension or rotation
	Local tenderness, radiation to arms, associated head injury
	Neurological assessment, e.g. myotomes, dermatomes; C3–C5 keep the diaphragm alive
	Radiographs (AP/odontoid, lateral, C1–C7 and top T1; swimmer's view if needed). CT/MRI as required
C1	Atlas (Jefferson) burst fracture, direct load to top of head
C2	Type I, II or III odontoid fracture; hangman's posterior fracture
C5/C6	Common position for fracture and/or subluxation
	Treatment is with immobilization; joint fusion for non-union
Thoracic	Types of injury: crush, burst, wedge fractures, T11–L1 dislocation
	Due to direct or indirect trauma; hyperflexion, extension or rotation
	Pathological bone, e.g. osteoporotic
	Local tenderness, paraplegia if unstable/displaced, associated head injury
	Full neurological assessment, e.g. myotomes, dermatomes
	Radiographs (AP, lateral). CT/MRI as required
	Treatment is with immobilization; fixation for instability
Lumbar	Types of injury: compression or transverse process fractures
	Pathological bone, e.g. osteoporotic
	Local tenderness, cauda equina syndrome if displaced (see spinal cord compression)
	Full neurological assessment, e.g. myotomes, dermatomes, saddle anaesthesia, per rectum examination
	Radiographs (AP, lateral). CT/MRI as required
	Treatment is with immobilization; fixation for instability or pathological fractures

* The acute management of all potential spinal injuries is airway with C-spine immobilization, followed by breathing, circulation and a full examination with log-roll (follow ATLS guidelines). The vast majority of fractures are treated conservatively with immobilization. Some suggest steroids as part of spinal injury treatment. Anterior cord syndrome (flexion/rotation injuries) is paraplegia with loss of temperature and pain sensation. Central cord syndrome (e.g. syringomelia) is motor loss in arms and legs (arms >> legs), with sacral sparing. Brown-Sequard syndrome is a hemisection of the cord with ipsilateral loss of power (paralysis) and proprioception, and loss of pain and temperature sensation on the contralateral side. Posterior cord syndrome (hyperextension injuries) is ataxia and loss of proprioception predominantly. The presence of a C-spine fracture increases the risk of fracture elsewhere in the spinal column.

Investigations and treatment
- As for back pain
- Surgery:
  — indicated for severe neurological presentations, e.g. progressive cervical myelopathy
  — decompression and spinal fusion.

SPINAL CORD COMPRESSION

Acute spinal cord compression is an emergency and may be associated with a variety of causes:

- Tumour (local or metastatic)
- Abscess, e.g. epidural abscess
- Trauma
- Disc prolapse (central)
- Tuberculosis.

Clinical presentation
- Bilateral leg pain
- Radicular (nerve root) pain at the compression level
- Paraesthesia below the compression level
- Upper and lower motor neurone signs dependent on the compression level
- Sphincter disturbance
- Cauda equina syndrome indicates lumbar (L1 and below) nerve root compression and results in characteristic lower motor neurone symptoms:
  — micturition disturbance with key features of hesitancy and urgency
  — faecal incontinence due to anal sphincter tone dysfunction
  — increasing motor weakness associated with gait disorder
  — saddle (perianal) anaesthesia.

Investigations
- Blood tests including serum B_{12}
- Lumbar puncture if not contraindicated
- Chest and plain spinal radiographs
- Spinal MRI.

Treatment
Management is determined by the cause and location of the lesion. The common therapeutic options are:

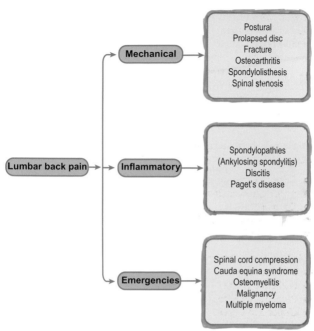

Figure 4.14 Classification of causes of lumbar back pain.

- High-dose i.v. corticosteroids, e.g. dexamethasone 8–16 mg
- Urgent surgical exploration with decompression or excision
- Chemotherapy or radiotherapy for malignant disease.

LUMBAR BACK PAIN

It is said that approximately 30% of UK homes have one adult or more who is in pain, with 25% of these households having two adults in that position. Back pain is an important cause of absenteeism from work and the cost of managing back pain and sciatica alone is approximately £6.3 billion/year. Lumbar back pain is simply a collective term for a group of conditions that present with this exceedingly common complaint.

Causes of back pain
See Figure 4.14.

Clinical presentation

The clinical presentation of mechanical and inflammatory conditions is somewhat similar. The differentiating factors are as follows:

- Age at onset:
  — <50 years: mechanical postural pain, prolapsed disc, spondylopathies
  — >50 years: degenerative condition, osteoporosis, malignancy.
- Rate of onset and the time of day the pain is most notable
- Unilateral or bilateral back and leg pain ≥ improves w/ AS.
- The presence of morning stiffness and the effect of exercise
- The presence of neurological symptoms and signs (emergency signs)
- Problems with bladder, bowel or sexual function (Potential emergency signs).

Investigations

- Blood tests including:
  — ESR may be increased in inflammatory back pain
  — bone screen for, e.g., multiple myeloma, Paget's disease
  — prostate specific antigen (PSA) if presentation suggests prostatic disease.
- Radiographs: disc space narrowing and joint arthritis
- MRI: indicated for neurological deficits and malignancy
- CT and bone scan: spondylolisthesis and some bone tumours, e.g. osteoid osteoma.

Treatment

- Conservative:
  — analgesics, e.g. NSAIDs
  — limited bed rest, though dependent on cause
  — physiotherapy.
- Surgical:
  — caudal or facet joint injections
  — spinal fusion on occasion.

PROLAPSED INTERVERTEBRAL DISC DISEASE

Prolapse involves nerve root compression due to posterolateral herniation of the nucleus pulposus through the annulus fibrosus, with a predisposition for the L4/L5/S1 region. It commonly occurs in males in their 3rd to 5th decade, long-distance drivers and heavy manual labourers. *Clinical presentation* is with back pain, referred leg pain and sciatica, with motor and sensory symptoms and signs over the distribution of the nerve root being irritated. Higher disc prolapses may affect the femoral nerve instead. Exacerbating factors are sitting, coughing and sneezing. Straight leg raise test positive for nerve root irritation. Diagnosis is confirmed with MRI. *Treatment* involves initial rest (avoid prolonged), analgesia, and physiotherapy. Surgery involves spinal discectomy.

SPONDYLOLISTHESIS

Spondylolisthesis is a slipping forward of one vertebral body onto the one below, often due to a congenital or trauma-induced defect of the pars interarticularis (ossification defect), with a predisposition for the L4/L5/S1 region. A pars defect without slip is more common and is known as spondylolysis. It commonly occurs in Caucasians, males, children and athletes (gymnasts), and is associated with other spinal pathology (scoliosis, kyphosis). *Clinical presentation* is with chronic back pain on standing and exercise. The exacerbating factor is spinal hyperextension, with movement and exercise sometimes restricted. Back pain, sciatica and radiculopathy are common. Diagnosis is confirmed with oblique radiographs ('Scottie dog' sign), CT or MRI. *Treatment* involves initial rest, analgesia and physiotherapy. Surgery, e.g. decompression and spinal fusion, is indicated for severe slips.

SPINAL STENOSIS

Stenosis (narrowing) of the spinal canal is most commonly due to degenerative changes and rarely due to prolapse, malignancy or congenital narrowing. *Clinical presentation* is of nerve root compression leading to neurological symptoms. Exacerbating factors are exercise and spinal extension, e.g. walking, leading to back pain referred to the buttocks and legs (spinal or neurogenic claudication); relief is achieved by spinal flexion and rest. Diagnosis is confirmed with CT or MRI, but remember to exclude vascular causes (peripheral vascular disease). *Treatment* involves lifestyle changes (weight loss), analgesia and physiotherapy. Surgery involves spinal decompression.

SCOLIOSIS

Scoliosis is a 3D lateral curvature of the thoracolumbar spine with rotational deformity of the vertebrae and ribs. The classification of scoliosis is:

- Postural: secondary to a pathology outwith the spine causing a mild scoliosis often seen in children or in pelvic obliquity; bending over abolishes the curve
- Structural: a fixed deformity from within the spine that does not change with posture.

The causes of scoliosis are:

- Congenital: bony irregularity leading to atypical spinal development, e.g. hemivertebrae, osteopathic scoliosis
- Idiopathic: seen in children of all ages, the cause is unknown, e.g. adolescent idiopathic scoliosis
- Secondary: rare primary cause leads to secondary curvature of the spine, e.g. leg length discrepancy, hip deformity
- Neuropathic: abnormal muscle spasm action leads to uneven forces on the spine, e.g. sciatica, cerebral palsy
- Degenerative: usually of the lumbar spine in the elderly.

Adolescent idiopathic scoliosis (AIS)

AIS is commonly seen before puberty, and ceases when growth comes to an end. It is characterized by lateral curvature of the thoracolumbar spine (>10°), with rotational deformity of the vertebrae and ribs (convex to right) causing a prominent hump on spine flexion. It is more common in girls, who are usually tall for their age. The younger the child and the greater the curve, the worse the prognosis.

Clinical presentation
- Peri-pubertal girls
- Spinal curve often first seen by parents
- One shoulder elevated above the other
- Decreased chest expansion.

Investigations
- Radiographs (PA and lateral of spine):
  — Cobb's angle is the maximum angle of curvature of the primary curve
  — repeat regularly to monitor progression.

- MRI:
  — plan surgery
  — possible associated spinal disorder.

Treatment
- Conservative:
  - physiotherapy
  - bracing for 30–40° curves with limited progression.
- Surgical:
  — indicated for severely progressing curves (>40°)
  — internal fixation and fusion.

BONE AND JOINT INFECTIONS

SEPTIC ARTHRITIS

Septic arthritis occurs when there is a bacterial infection of the joint. It is a surgical emergency. Untreated septic arthritis can rapidly (within hours) cause joint destruction due to release of proteolytic enzymes which degrade bone, cartilage and soft tissues. The incidence is 2–10/100 000 but septic arthritis is more common in patients with arthroplasty and coexisting joint diseases such as RA. Joints of the lower limb are most frequently affected and the hip (most common in infants) and knee (most common in children and adults) are the commonest sites. However, any joint, and sometimes more than one joint, can be affected.

Pathogenesis
The disease usually occurs as the result of bacterial spread from another site. The most common primary sites of infection are:

- The skin, possibly compromised due to trauma, e.g. cellulitis or surgery
- Neighbouring bone (e.g. in osteomyelitis)
- Haematogenous spread (e.g. respiratory or urinary tract infection).

The organisms most commonly implicated include:

- *Staphylococcus aureus*
- Gram-negative bacilli (in diabetics, the elderly or i.v. drug users)
- *Neisseria gonorrhoeae* (sexually active young adults)

● *Haemophilus influenzae* (neonates and infants)
● *Staphylococcus epidermidis* (especially in joint replacements).

Other *risk factors* include:

- Extremes of age
- Poverty and malnourishment, e.g. in the developing nations
- Immunosuppression, e.g. HIV/AIDS, steroids, IVDU
- Diabetes mellitus.

Clinical presentation
● Acute onset of a painful, red, hot and swollen joint
● Muscle spasm leading to immobility of joint (pseudoparesis)
● Systemic upset: tachycardia, fever, malaise, anorexia
● Atypical presentation may occur in the elderly, the immunosuppressed or those with established joint disease
● Polyarthralgia, tenosynovitis, urogenital symptoms and a pustular rash may occur in *N. gonorrhoeae* infection
● A chronic infection in a total joint replacement may result in loosening of the implant. This may be the sole clinical feature of infection.

Investigations
- Blood tests:
  — haematology: raised ESR and WCC
  — biochemistry: raised CRP.
- Joint aspiration before antibiotics given (see Table 3.3):
  — turbid fluid with raised WCC
  — organism may be demonstrated by microscopy and Gram staining or isolated by culture.
- Microbiology:
  — obtain blood cultures and/or cultures from possible sites of primary infection (wound site, urogenital system, chest).
- Imaging:
  — radiographs: joint effusion, soft tissue swelling
  — USS: may aid diagnostic aspiration.
- MRI has a high sensitivity and specificity.

Treatment
● Resuscitation as necessary and high-dose i.v. antibiotics:
  — benzyl penicillin and flucloxacillin, for 2–3 weeks, followed by oral therapy (total duration or treatment ~6 weeks)
  — other antibiotics may be indicated depending on results of culture and sensitivity testing.

- Analgesics or NSAIDs for pain relief
- Non-pharmacological approaches:
  — joint incision and drainage with lavage is the gold standard
  — joint immobilization followed by physiotherapy
  — repeated joint aspiration
  — removal of infected implant material.

Prognosis

The prognosis is good with appropriate treatment but complications may occur including:

- Septic shock
- Abscess or sinus formation
- Joint destruction, periarticular osteoporosis, ankylosis and secondary OA
- Avascular necrosis
- Inhibition of limb growth and deformity (with growth plate involvement in children).

OSTEOMYELITIS

Osteomyelitis is infection of the bone. In children it commonly occurs at the metaphysis close to the epiphyseal plate whereas in adults any site in the bone may be affected. Spread of infection to bone occurs via: (1) blood-borne spread from the skin or respiratory, gastrointestinal or genitourinary tract; or (2) direct spread post trauma (including surgery). Initial infection and inflammation of the metaphysis lead to lifting and removal of the periosteum due to a subperiosteal abscess, leading eventually to original bone death (sequestrum) due to a compromised blood supply causing necrosis (cortex infarction), with new bone formation as a consequence (involucrum). Common infecting organisms are:

- *Staphylococcus aureus*
- *Streptococcus pneumoniae* or *Streptococcus pyogenes*
- *Salmonella* (associated with patients who have sickle cell disease)
- *Haemophilus influenzae* and haemolytic streptococci (children).

Risk factors

- Extremes of age
- Immunosuppression (e.g. HIV, AIDS, steroids, IVDU)
- Diabetes mellitus

- Joint replacement
- Trauma.

Clinical presentation

- Pain, tenderness, warmth and redness over affected bone
- Vertebrae can be affected in adults
- Effusions of nearby joint
- Systemic upset: fever, malaise, anorexia, weight loss.

Investigations

- Blood tests:
  — haematology: raised ESR and WCC
  — biochemistry: raised CRP.
- Microbiology:
  — culture of affected site
  — blood cultures or culture from site of primary infection (e.g. skin, wound, urogenital tract) before antibiotics given.
- Imaging:
  — radiographs initially normal, but after 2 weeks osteolysis, metaphyseal rarefaction, and subsequently periosteal elevation and bone formation, osteosclerosis and cortical thickening possible
  — MRI has a high sensitivity and specificity.

Treatment

- Resuscitation and high-dose i.v. antibiotics:
  — benzyl penicillin and flucloxacillin, for 2–3 weeks, followed by oral therapy, aiming for a total duration of treatment of 6 weeks
  — other antibiotics may be indicated depending on results of culture and sensitivity testing.
- Analgesics or NSAIDs for pain relief
- Non-pharmacological approaches:
  — immobilization will help prevent contracture
  — physiotherapy.
- Surgery:
  — surgical drainage with removal of dead bone and tissue.

Prognosis

Good with appropriate treatment but several complications may occur including:

- Septic arthritis
- Bone deformity and growth disturbance
- Fracture (pathological)

- Chronic osteomyelitis and/or recurrence
- Abscess formation.

NB: Brodie's abscess is a less severe form of osteomyelitis where natural defences have partially overcome the infection, leading to an abscess confined within cortical/sclerotic bone (in the metaphysis). This appears as a halo on MRI. This type of abscess is commonly associated with distal femoral and tibial injuries.

CHRONIC OSTEOMYELITIS

Chronic osteomyelitis is a persistent bone infection which sometimes follows acute osteomyelitis (due to persistent infection/ poor antibiotic delivery to necrotic bone or antibiotic-resistant microorganisms), particularly in patients with prosthetic implants or those with metalwork in place after (open) fracture fixation. The Cierny-Mader classification can be used for chronic osteomyelitis.

Clinical presentation
- Pain, swelling and redness over affected site (e.g. long bones)
- Sinus, ulcer or abscess development
- Systemic upset, weight loss and fever
- Risk factors are similar to those for acute osteomyelitis.

Investigations
- Blood tests:
  — haematology: raised ESR and WCC
  — biochemistry: raised CRP.
- Microbiology:
  — blood cultures and cultures from affected site or likely primary site (a bone biopsy may be needed).
- Imaging:
  — radiographs show osteosclerosis, cortical thickening, periosteal reaction and areas of osteolysis
  — CT and/or MRI will help differentiate soft tissue infection and necrotic bone.

Treatment
- Long-term antibiotic treatment, choice culture dependent
- Pain relief with analgesics e.g. NSAIDs
- Lifestyle changes, e.g. stop smoking, better nutrition
- Immobilization with splint or plaster

- Surgery:
  — drainage ± dead bone removal with external fixation
  — removal of implants or metalwork
  — amputation rarely indicated.

Prognosis
Various complications may occur:

- Pathological fracture
- Secondary amyloidosis
- Squamous cell carcinoma of sinus and surrounding skin (Marjolin's ulcer).

VIRAL ARTHRITIS

Viral infection may be associated with an acute, but self-limiting, form of arthritis. Viruses which have been implicated include:

- Hepatitis B and C
- HIV (also can be associated with chronic polyarthralgia)
- Chickenpox
- Mumps
- Erythrovirus (formerly parvovirus) B19
- Rubella.

Clinical presentation
- Acute polyarthritis with a variable distribution
- History of recent 'viral' illness
- Fever or rash.

Investigations
- Microbiology:
  — IgM antibodies to offending pathogen on serological testing.

Management
- NSAIDs/analgesics
- Most cases are self-limiting.

BONE TUMOURS

Osteoid osteoma is a benign bone-forming tumour of young males, often localising to the shaft of the major long bones and spine. The clinical and histological presentation of an *osteoblastoma* is similar, and some argue it is a large osteoid osteoma. *Clinical presentation* is with a severe dull pain, which is worse at night and relieved by NSAIDs (often aspirin). *Diagnosis* is with a radiograph (sclerosis with a radiolucent nidus) and CT/bone scan with bone biopsy. *Treatment* is with excision if prominent symptoms are present.

Osteochondroma is a very common cartilage tumour of children and adolescents, often localizing to the metaphyses of the major long bones. It forms from anomalous cartilage found on the outer surface of the growth plate; endochondral ossification under the cartilage may result in sessile (flattened) or pedunculated (stalked) bony lesions covered with hyaline cartilage. An autosomal dominant multiple form exists. *Clinical presentation* is rare as most give no symptoms. Pain and tingling may occur due to strain on nearby vessels and nerves. *Diagnosis* is with radiograph (bony outgrowth seen) or CT/MRI. *Treatment* is often unnecessary, with excision indicated only if prominent symptoms are present. Malignant transformation is infrequent and is commoner with multiple lesions.

Enchondroma is a common cartilage tumour in adults, often localizing within the metaphysis of long bones, e.g. femur, but also within the small bones of the hand. *Clinical presentation* is rare as most give no symptoms. Pain and swelling may occur due to large tumours. *Diagnosis* is with radiograph (oval lytic regions, calcification). *Treatment* is often unnecessary, with curettage (scraping-out) indicated if prominent symptoms or fracture are present. Malignant transformation is infrequent but regular radiographs are necessary to confirm resolution. A multiple form is known as Ollier's disease.

Osteosarcoma is a very rare, but the most common, malignant bone tumour of children and adults (bi-modal), particularly males (~1.5:1). It is associated with retinoblastoma, Paget's disease and radiation. Localization is often in the metaphyses of the long bones (e.g. femur, tibia, humerus), often leading to bone destruction. Blood-borne metastases may occur in the lung. *Clinical presentation* is often with bone pain, swelling and erythema, with a possible mass felt. Respiratory symptoms, e.g. cough, if lung invasion. *Diagnosis* is with radiograph (lytic sclerosis, Codman's triangle, sunray spicules, bone destruction) and bloods ($\uparrow$ ESR, $\uparrow$ ALP). Bone biopsy is mandatory. CT of the chest for metastases is often necessary. *Treatment* is chemotherapy, e.g. doxorubicin, followed by excision and joint arthroplasty. Amputation is possible. 5-year survival = 60–70% with modern chemotherapy.

Giant cell tumours (osteoclastomas) are locally aggressive and recurrent tumours of young adults (20–40 yrs), often localising to the epiphysis of long bones, particularly near the knee. Metastases are rare, often late, and commonly occur in the lungs. *Diagnosis* is with a radiograph (non-sclerotic, expanding lytic/cystic lesions, 'soap bubble' appearance) and MRI with bone biopsy. CXR and CT chest are used to detect metastases. *Treatment* is with excision.

Myeloma is the most frequently seen primary bone tumour, arising from the proliferation of plasma cells (B cells). It often is seen in those >50 yrs, peaking at 65–70 yrs. Multiple myeloma with widespread metastases is common. *Clinical presentation* can be with pain (ribs/spine/fracture), anaemia, infection and/or renal failure. *Diagnosis* is with bloods ($\downarrow$Hb, $\uparrow$ESR, $\uparrow$Ca^{2+}, $\uparrow$immunoglobulin, $\uparrow$urea and creatinine), urine (Bence-Jones protein), a radiograph (punched-out lesions), MRI and a bone marrow biopsy. *Treatment* can be curative with bone marrow transplant +/– chemotherapy. Symptomatic treatment includes bisphosphonates, radiotherapy and fixation (bone pain/fracture), erythropoietin (anaemia) and dialysis (renal failure).

Ewing's sarcoma is a very rare, but extremely malignant, small round cell bone tumour of children and young adults. Localization is usually in the diaphysis of long and flat bones, e.g. femur, pelvis or spine, frequently leading to bone destruction. Blood-borne metastases often occur to the lung, liver and other parts of the skeleton. *Clinical presentation* is often with bone pain, swelling and tenderness, possibly with fever. *Diagnosis* is with radiograph (lytic lesions, soft tissue swelling, 'onion-skin' new bone), bloods ($\uparrow$WCC) and bone biopsy (pustular appearance). A characteristic translocation is found on cytogenetic analysis – t(11;22). CT of the chest for metastases is often necessary. *Treatment* is chemotherapy, e.g. etoposide, and either radiotherapy or excision. Amputation may be required. 5-year survival = 50–75% with modern chemotherapy.

Chondrosarcoma is a rare malignant tumour of bone affecting older people and mainly the metaphyses of long bone, pelvis, shoulder girdle and spine. Histological grades I–III are seen. Surgical resection is the mainstay of treatment as there is no response to chemotherapy or radiotherapy.

Secondary bone tumours often metastasize from the prostate, breast, kidney, lung, thyroid or skin. Patients present with symptoms from their primary lesion, along with a spectrum of malaise, bone pain, pathological fracture (risk assessment done using the Mirels scoring system) and spinal cord compression. Radiographs and blood tests (see Table 3.2) are necessary. Further imaging and bone biopsy will often be needed. Analgesia, bisphosphonates, radiotherapy and chemotherapy, along with surgery for cord decompression or to stabilize actual or impending pathological fractures, are the possible management avenues.

NERVE INJURY

GRADES OF NERVE INJURY

- Ischaemia (transient nerve ischaemia; lasts seconds to minutes)
- Neuropraxia (local demyelination; recovery 1–3 weeks)
- Axonotmesis (nerve axon death, nerve tube intact; recovery 1–3 mm/24 h)
- Neurotmesis (nerve axon death, nerve tube transected or crushed; recovery 1–3 mm/24 h but incomplete even with surgery).

Clinical assessment with neurophysiological studies will often provide a definitive diagnosis.

BRACHIAL PLEXUS INJURY

Injury to the brachial plexus commonly follows a traction injury that forces the shoulder and neck apart, or one that pulls the arm upwards. Both types of injury are possible with complicated vaginal deliveries e.g. breech birth. High-energy trauma (may damage entire brachial plexus) or severely displaced pectoral girdle fractures are more common precipitants in adults. Radiographs (C-spine and CXR) with MRI of the C-spine will aid diagnosis.

Common clinical presentation
- C5/C6/C7 root affected (Erb's paralysis)
  — Arm adducted, forearm pronated, palm upwards and backwards (waiter's tip position)
- T1 root affected (similar presentation to ulnar nerve injury)
  — Claw hand as intrinsic muscles of hand affected
  — Sensory loss in T1 dermatome distribution
  — Associated with Horner's syndrome, Pancoast's tumour, and a cervical rib

AXILLARY NERVE INJURY

Injury to the axillary nerve most commonly occurs following an anterior shoulder dislocation or a proximal humeral fracture (when the axillary nerve passes around the surgical neck of the humerus).

Clinical presentation

- Paraesthesia or sensory loss over the lateral aspect of the upper arm – 'regimental badge sign'
- Shoulder abduction predominantly lost due to paralysis of deltoid muscle.

RADIAL NERVE INJURY

Injury (see Chapter 7) or compression of the radial nerve most commonly occurs as it passes around the spinal groove of humerus or into the supinator muscle. A neuropraxia can occur due to compression in the axilla either due to axillary crutches or when an intoxicated person passes out with an arm draping over a chair – 'Saturday Night Palsy'. Isolated posterior interosseous injury may occur (see Chapter 7).

Clinical presentation

- Paralysis of the wrist, thumb and finger extensors, leading to wrist drop and decreased grip strength. A higher lesion will affect elbow extension also
- Forearm or triceps muscle wasting possible
- Sensory loss of a small area of the dorsum of the hand, i.e. 1st web space, or the posterior forearm if a higher lesion.
- Posterior interosseous injury alone will preserve wrist extention

Treatment
- Conservative:
  — physiotherapy and wrist splints may help
- Surgical:
  — nerve grafting or tendon transposition.

ULNAR NERVE INJURY

Injury (see Chapter 7) or compression of the ulnar nerve most commonly occurs as it passes posteriorly around the medial condyle of the elbow and through the cubital tunnel, or as it travels adjacent to the hook of hamate in the wrist in Guyon's canal,

Risk factors for compression
Pregnancy, RA or OA leading to bony deformity at the elbow e.g. cubitus valgus, myxoedema, elbow or hook of hamate fracture, elbow dislocation, repeated pressure at the elbow or wrist, or ganglion.

Clinical presentation
- Pain and paraesthesia of the medial side of the elbow with radiation to the ulnar distribution (sensory loss in little finger and ulnar half of ring finger)
- Hypothenar, lumbrical and interosseous muscle wasting with paralysis leading to finger muscle weakness and hand clawing (higher lesions e.g. at the elbow, lead to radial deviation of the hand)
- Tardy ulnar nerve palsy: slow onset post injury (years) that is often associated with cubitus valgus.

Treatment
Corticosteroid injection or decompression with anterior transposition at the elbow for compressive symptoms.

MEDIAN NERVE INJURY

Injury (see Chapter 7) or compression (see Carpal Tunnel Syndrome) of the median nerve can occur. With trauma it is most common following an elbow fracture, forearm fracture (anterior interosseous nerve) or wrist fractures lacerations.

Clinical presentation
- High lesion/injury e.g. at the elbow
  — Paralysis of pronation, wrist palmarflexion, thumb IPJ flexion
  — Muscle wasting of lateral aspect of forearm
  — Sensory loss of the lateral palm and radial three and half digits (preserved with anterior interosseous injury)
- Low lesion/injury e.g. at the wrist (see Carpal Tunnel Syndrome)
  — Thenar muscle and radial two lumbrical paralysis +/− atrophy
  — Sensory loss of the radial three and half digits

SCIATIC NERVE INJURY

Injury to the sciatic nerve can occur following a posterior hip dislocation or following a pelvic fracture.

Clinical presentation
- Sensory loss below the knee:
  — saphenous nerve distribution spared (see Figure 1.19)
- Paralysis of the hamstrings and the muscles below the knee joint.

TIBIAL NERVE INJURY

Injury to the tibial nerve can occur following a fracture of the tibial shaft or the medial malleolus, or following excessive external pressure, e.g. tight plaster cast, compartment syndrome.

Clinical presentation
- Sensory loss over the sole of the foot
- Foot plantar and toe flexion paralysis with muscle wasting in the sole of the foot if chronic
- Toe clawing possible.

COMMON PERONEAL NERVE INJURY

Injury (see Chapter 7) or compression of the peroneal nerve as it passes around the fibula neck occurs following a fracture of the fibula neck, or following excessive external pressure, e.g. plaster cast, ganglion of the proximal tibiofibular joint.

Clinical presentation
- Foot drop due to paralysis of dorsiflexion (deep peroneal nerve) and eversion (superficial peroneal nerve), leading to unopposed plantarflexion and foot inversion
- High-stepping gait
- Sensory loss of the central dorsum of the foot and the lower lateral aspect of the leg (see Figure 1.19)

Treatment
- Conservative:
  — physiotherapy +/− foot-drop splints.
- Surgical: decompression if compression evident.

HIP AND KNEE ARTHROPLASTY

Arthroplasty, meaning 'joint changes shape', is the repair or replacement of part, or all, of a particular joint in the body, such as the hip or knee. There are many different types of arthroplasty (excision, resurfacing, hemi, total), with replacement arthroplasty the one most commonly used within the UK.

Common indications

- Osteoarthritis, e.g. of the hip or knee (pain at night +/- refractory to analgesia)
- Certain fractures e.g. some fractures of the proximal humerus or femur
- Rheumatoid arthritis
- Late complication of paediatric hip disorders (DDH, Perthes, SUFE)
- Avascular necrosis.

Complications

- Prolonged pain commoner with knee arthroplasty
- Leg length discrepancy with hip arthroplasty (15%)
- Infection:
  - 1–3% of cases, more common in knee arthroplasty than hip
  - Common organisms are coagulase-negative staphylococci (Staphylococcus epidermidis) and coagulase-positive staphylococci (Staphylococcus aureus)
  - Early prosthetic loosening can occur
  - Treatment can range from antibiotics to excision arthroplasty (e.g. Girdlestone's for an infected hip prosthesis) or even amputation
  - Prevention is best practice via dedicated elective orthopaedic wards, aseptic and precise surgical techniques, laminar flow operating theatres and peri-operative antibiotics.
- Aseptic loosening
- Dislocation of the hip (10%)
- Peri-prosthetic fracture
- General medical complications (see Chapter 7):
  - infection, e.g. LRTI or UTI
  - MI/DVT/PE (DVT prophylaxis is essential).
- Death (0.5%–1%).

CHAPTER 5

RHEUMATOLOGY

RHEUMATOID ARTHRITIS

Rheumatoid arthritis (RA) is the most common form of inflammatory arthritis. It affects all ethnic groups and the peak incidence is in women between the ages of 30 and 50 years. The prevalence in Caucasians is about 1% and the female:male ratio is 3:1.

Pathogenesis

The pathogenesis of RA is incompletely understood, but it is currently thought that genetically susceptible individuals develop the disease in response to an unidentified possibly infectious trigger, which induces immune activation and cross-reactivity with endogenous antigens, leading to chronic inflammation in the joints and other tissues. Females are more susceptible than males and the disease remits during pregnancy. There is a strong genetic association with HLA-DR4 and DR1, but other genetic variants also contribute. Smoking is associated with more severe disease.

Clinical features

The characteristic clinical features of RA are:

- Symmetrical joint pain, stiffness and swelling affecting the small joints of the hands and feet, wrists and other joints (Figure 5.1)
- Early morning stiffness >1 hour
- Synovial swelling and hypertrophy with an infiltrate of inflammatory cells including lymphocytes, plasma cells and macrophages
- Periarticular osteoporosis, bone erosions and cartilage erosions with progressive joint damage and destruction (Figure 5.2)
- A clinical course of exacerbation and remissions
- Extra-articular and systemic features including:
  — fever, fatigue, weight loss
  — vasculitis and rheumatoid nodules
  — scleritis, keratoconjunctivitis
  — dry eyes and dry mouth (Sjögren's syndrome)
  — pericarditis, pleurisy
  — pulmonary fibrosis, lung nodules
  — anaemia
  — amyloidosis
  — Felty's syndrome (splenomegaly, leucopenia, lymphadenopathy, anaemia, thrombocytopenia).

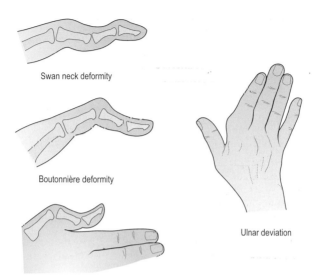

Swan neck deformity

Boutonnière deformity

Z-shaped thumb

Ulnar deviation

Figure 5.1 Deformities seen in rheumatoid hands. Ulnar and volar deviation of the finger joints due to synovial inflammation of the wrist and MCPJs. Wrist subluxation may lead to a prominent ulnar styloid. Tendon rupture, secondary to swelling of tendon sheaths and/or reported frictional trauma, can occur, e.g. extensors, FPL. Swan neck deformity is due to PIPJ hyperextension, with MCPJ and DIPJ flexion. FDS rupture or extensor digitorum shortening will lead to a similar presentation. Boutonnière deformity is due to a deficiency of the extensor tendon central slip leading to DIPJ hyperextension and PIPJ flexion.

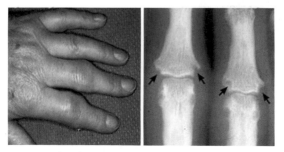

Figure 5.2 RA of the hands. Distinctive changes on radiographs include soft tissue swelling, periarticular osteoporosis, symmetrical joint space narrowing, juxta-articular erosions (black arrows) and joint subluxation/dislocation leading to deformity.

Investigations
- Blood tests:
  — haematology: normochromic normocytic anaemia, thrombocytosis, raised ESR with active disease
  — biochemistry: raised CRP, abnormal LFTs with active disease
  — immunology: RF positive (75%), anti-CCP antibody positive (70%), ANA positive (50%) (see Chapter 3).
- Joint aspiration:
  — sterile, cloudy fluid with raised WCC and low viscosity.
- Imaging:
  — periarticular osteoporosis, bone erosions and joint space narrowing on radiographs (Figure 5.2)
  — systemic osteoporosis and fractures
  — osteoporosis on DEXA.

Treatment
- DMARDs (see Chapter 8):
  — early use protects against irreversible joint damage
  — methotrexate or sulfasalazine generally used as first choice; combination therapy is used for resistant disease.
- Corticosteroids (see Chapter 8):
  — intermittent steroid injections for disease flares
  — low-dose oral steroids as adjunct to DMARD therapy.
- Biological therapy (see Chapter 8):
  — anti-TNF therapy for resistant disease
  — anti-B cell therapy for RA resistant to anti-TNF therapy.
- Intra-articular steroid injections for problem joints
- NSAIDs/analgesics for pain relief
- Non-pharmacological approaches:
  — education, joint protection
  — splints, appliances and household aids
  — rest during disease flares
  — physiotherapy.
- Surgery indicated for progressive disease resistant to medical management:
  — tendon repair
  — synovectomy
  — joint replacement surgery
  — arthrodesis and osteotomy.

Prognosis
- Half have radiological signs of erosions and joint space narrowing within 2 years

- Life expectancy is decreased (~10 years for women, ~4 years for men), due mainly to an increased risk of cardiovascular disease
- Favourable prognostic signs are:
  — male
  — late-onset joint erosion
  — lack of extra-articular features
  — low levels of RF and CRP.

SERONEGATIVE SPONDYLOARTHRITIS

This group of inflammatory joint disorders has overlapping clinical features. These disorders differ from RA in that:

- Serological tests for RF are negative
- Joint involvement is mostly asymmetrical
- Inflammation occurs at sites of tendon insertions (enthesopathy) and in fibrocartilaginous joints (sacroiliitis and spondylitis)
- New bone formation is a prominent feature
- There is a strong genetic association with HLA-B27
- Extra-articular features differ from RA.

ANKYLOSING SPONDYLITIS

Ankylosing spondylitis (AS) is a chronic inflammatory disorder characterized by inflammation of the sacroiliac joints and spine leading ultimately to spinal fusion. The onset is usually during young adulthood (age 20–30) and the disease is more common in men (3:1). The overall prevalence is about 0.15% and more than 90% are positive for the HLA-B27 antigen.

Pathogenesis
The pathogenesis of AS is incompletely understood, but it is currently thought that genetically susceptible individuals develop the disease in response to an unidentified infectious trigger, which induces immune activation and cross-reactivity with endogenous antigens in fibrocartilaginous and synovial joints leading to chronic inflammation.

Risk factors
- Genetic: strong association with HLA-B27
- Hormonal: males more susceptible than females.

Clinical features

- Early-morning lower back pain and stiffness for >3 months, which improves with exercise
- Diminished range of spinal movement in all directions leading to characteristic posture:
  - loss of lumbar lordosis
  - stooped posture
  - hyperextension of neck
  - flexion at hips and knees.
- Diminished chest expansion
- Plantar fasciitis, Achilles tendonitis
- Extra-articular features:
  - anterior uveitis
  - aortic incompetence
  - restrictive ventilatory defect.

Investigations

- Blood tests:
  - haematology: FBC usually normal, raised ESR with active disease
  - biochemistry: raised CRP with active disease
  - immunology: RF and ANA negative.
- Joint aspiration:
  - sterile, cloudy fluid with raised WCC and low viscosity.
- Imaging:
  - erosion, sclerosis and narrowing of sacroiliac joint on radiograph (MRI more sensitive in early disease)
  - ligament calcification in spine (syndesmophytes) with bony ankylosis in advanced disease
  - squaring of anterior vertebral bodies
  - vertebral fractures common.

Treatment

- Pain relief:
  - NSAIDs and analgesics.
- Non-pharmacological treatment:
  - physiotherapy, education, back exercises.
- Biological therapies (see Chapter 8):
  - anti-TNF therapy for resistant disease.
- DMARDs:
  - help peripheral joint disease but ineffective in spinal disease.
- Steroids:
  - systemic steroids for uveitis, local steroids for plantar fasciitis.

- Surgery:
  — joint replacement
  — spine osteotomy for severe deformity (rarely indicated).

Prognosis
- Generally good
- Most patients (75%) remain in employment
- Life span normal.

PSORIATIC ARTHRITIS

Psoriatic arthritis (PsA) is an inflammatory joint disease that occurs in association with psoriasis. The arthritis usually occurs after the onset of psoriasis (70%) but can antedate the skin disease (25%), and rarely presents at the same time (5%). About 7% of patients with psoriasis develop arthritis and it is associated with nail dystrophy and pitting. The overall population prevalence is about 0.1% and the peak age at onset is between 25 and 40. Males and females are affected equally.

Pathogenesis
The pathogenesis of PsA is unclear but, like other inflammatory joint diseases, it is thought to be caused by an infectious or other environmental trigger in a genetically susceptible individual.

Clinical presentation
A variety of presentations are recognized:

- Asymmetrical oligoarthritis (40%): large joint inflammatory arthritis often with involvement of PIP and DIP joints of the hands and feet
- Symmetrical polyarthritis (25%): clinically similar to RA, but nodules and serological features of RA absent
- Phalangeal arthritis (15%): typically affects men and predominantly targets the DIP joints; strongly associated with nail dystrophy
- Psoriatic spondylitis: similar to AS with or without peripheral joint involvement in one or more of the patterns described above
- Extra-articular features include:
  — uveitis
  — psoriatic skin rash
  — nail pitting and nail dystrophy.

Investigations
- Blood tests:
  — haematology: often normal; normochromic normocytic anaemia, thrombocytosis and raised ESR with active disease
  — biochemistry: raised CRP with active disease
  — immunology: RF, CCP antibodies and ANA negative (see Chapter 3).
- Joint aspiration:
  — sterile, cloudy fluid with raised WCC and low viscosity.
- Imaging:
  — bone erosions and joint space narrowing (Figure 5.2)
  — sacroiliitis.

Treatment
- DMARDs (see Chapter 8):
  — early use protects against irreversible joint damage
  — methotrexate is first choice (helps skin and joints); combination therapy is used for resistant disease
  — hydroxychloroquine used less often in case it causes flare in skin disease.
- Corticosteroids (see Chapter 8):
  — intermittent steroid injections for disease flares
  — low-dose oral steroids as adjunct to DMARD therapy.
- Biological therapy (see Chapter 8):
  — anti-TNF therapy for resistant disease.
- Intra-articular steroid injections for problem joints
- Pain relief (see Chapter 8):
  — NSAIDs and/or analgesics.
- Non-pharmacological treatment:
  — education, joint protection
  — splints, appliances and household aids
  — rest during disease flares
  — physiotherapy.
- Surgery indicated for progressive disease resistant to medical management:
  — synovectomy
  — joint replacement surgery
  — arthrodesis and osteotomy.

REACTIVE ARTHRITIS

Reactive arthritis is an acute inflammatory arthritis which typically affects large joints in an asymmetrical pattern. It may occur as part of Reiter's triad of arthritis, urethritis and conjunctivitis (Reiter's syndrome, Figure 5.3). Young men are predominantly affected (male:female 15:1) and typical onset is between 15 and 40 years. The population prevalence is about 0.016%.

Pathogenesis
The condition is thought to be caused by an infectious trigger in a genetically susceptible individual. This induces immune activation and cross-reactivity with endogenous antigens leading to acute inflammation in the joints and other affected tissues. Recognized triggers include *Salmonella, Shigella, Campylobacter* and *Yersinia,* or sexually acquired infection with *Chlamydia.*

Clinical presentation
- Acute asymmetrical large joint arthritis (often lower limbs)
- Heel pain, plantar fasciitis and Achilles tendonitis
- Conjunctivitis (30%)
- Urethritis, circinate balanitis (ulcers and vesicles surrounding the glans penis)
- Mouth ulcers
- Uveitis – anterior (iritis)
- Nail dystrophy and keratoderma blennorrhagica (lesions similar to pustular psoriasis develop on soles and palms).

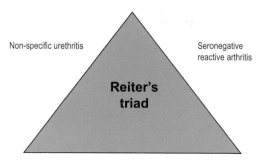

Figure 5.3 Although rare, Reiter's syndrome follows a genitourinary (*Chlamydia* or gonococcal infection following sexual transmission) or gastrointestinal (dysentery due to bacteria such as *Salmonella, Shigella*) infection, and presents with a triad of complaints.

Investigations
- Blood tests:
  — haematology: thrombocytosis and raised ESR
  — biochemistry: raised CRP
  — immunology: RF, ANA and CCP negative.
- Joint aspiration:
  — sterile, cloudy fluid with raised WCC and low viscosity
  — giant macrophages (Reiter cells) may be seen.
- Microbiology:
  — urine or stool culture for pathogens.
- Imaging:
  — periostitis of foot bones and pelvis, calcaneal spurs
  — sacroiliitis.

Treatment
- Corticosteroids (see Chapter 8):
  — intra-articular steroids, when infection excluded
  — short course of oral steroids.
- Pain relief (see Chapter 8):
  — NSAIDs/analgesics.
- DMARDs (see Chapter 8):
  — indicated for persistent or refractory disease
  — methotrexate and sulfasalazine usually used as first choice.
- Antibiotics:
  — tetracycline for *Chlamydia* urethritis.

Prognosis
- Generally good; 80% resolve within a year.
  ⤷ remaining 20% chronic, remitting, disabling disease.

ENTEROPATHIC ARTHRITIS

Approximately 15% of patients with IBD develop ankylosing spondylitis and/or a large joint asymmetrical peripheral inflammatory arthritis. If spine disease predominates, management is as described for AS; if peripheral disease predominates, management is as described for PsA.

SYSTEMIC VASCULITIS

The systemic vasculitides are a heterogeneous group of disorders characterized by inflammation and necrosis of blood vessel walls and organ damage. Vasculitis can occur in isolation or in association with other disorders such as RA and SLE. There are 100 new cases of primary vasculitis per million each year, most of which are giant cell arteritis. The vasculitides are commonly classified according to the Chapel Hill criteria, which separates the various types of vasculitis into whether small, medium or large vessels are affected, although this has limited clinical value in terms of prognosis and treatment. Here the different subtypes will be grouped according to the clinical features and management.

GIANT CELL ARTERITIS AND POLYMYALGIA RHEUMATICA

Giant cell arteritis (GCA) is the most common primary vasculitis. It typically affects medium-sized vessels in the head and neck, including the ophthalmic and temporal arteries. It is frequently associated with polymyalgia rheumatica (PMR) in which there is pain and stiffness affecting the proximal shoulder and pelvic girdle. Many patients who initially present with PMR go on to develop GCA; as such, these two conditions can be considered to be overlapping disorders. Both GCA and PMR are rare under the age of 55 years and the peak age of onset is about 70 years. The incidence of GCA is about 0.03% and the disease is more common in females (~3:1). PMR = joint pain. muscular pain suggestive of polymyositis

Pathogenesis
The cause of GCA and PMR is unknown but the disease is characterized by an inflammatory infiltrate of the affected vessels with destruction of the internal elastic lamina, granuloma formation and giant cell infiltration. Lesions are patchy in nature and affect only parts of the vessel wall (skip lesions).

Clinical presentation
- Headache
- Tenderness over temple or scalp
- Temporal artery swelling and tenderness, with loss of pulsation
- Facial pain and jaw claudication
- Proximal muscle pain and stiffness affecting pelvic and shoulder girdle (PMR)
- Visual disturbance, e.g. diplopia, amaurosis fugax
- Blindness due to involvement of ophthalmic, retinal and posterior ciliary arteries
- Systemic upset: fever, fatigue, malaise, anorexia, weight loss.

Investigations
- Blood tests:
  — haematology: normochromic normocytic anaemia, thrombocytosis, raised ESR
  — biochemistry: raised CRP, mildly abnormal LFTs
  — immunology: autoantibody screen negative.
- Biopsy:
  — temporal artery biopsy can confirm, but negative biopsy cannot exclude diagnosis due to skip lesions.
- Imaging:
  — DEXA to assess need for osteoporosis prophylaxis.
  ↳ steroid-induced.

Treatment
- Steroids are the treatment of choice for GCA and PMR:
  — initially, high-dose prednisolone (40–80 mg/24 h) for 4–6 weeks
  — reduce by 5 mg every 2–4 weeks according to response of symptoms and ESR
  — when dose of 15 mg is reached, reduce by 1–2 mg/month
  — most patients require 1–2 years of steroid therapy.
- Cytotoxics:
  — azathioprine and methotrexate are used as steroid-sparing agents in patients where unacceptably high doses of steroids are required to control the disease.

Prognosis
- Generally good; most patients respond well to treatment, but steroid-induced osteoporosis is a common complication unless prophylaxis is given (see Chapter 8).

POLYARTERITIS NODOSA, MICROSCOPIC POLYANGIITIS AND CHURG–STRAUSS SYNDROME

Polyarteritis nodosa (PAN) mostly affects men between the ages of 30 and 50 years. It is characterized by vessel wall necrosis and aneurysm formation, leading to thrombosis and infarction. It is often associated with HBV infection. Clinical presentation is with systemic upset (fever, weight loss, lethargy, myalgia, arthralgia), peripheral neuropathy (mononeuritis multiplex), GI pain and bleeding (mucosa ulceration and infarction), acute renal failure and hypertension, skin ulceration and rash (gangrene, nodules), and cardiac disease (MI, cardiac failure, pericarditis). Investigations show anaemia with an increased ESR and CRP, whilst angiography of renal, coeliac and hepatic arteries may show microaneurysms. Immunology screen typically shows a positive ANCA and reduced complement levels. Organ biopsy may be helpful in making a diagnosis.

Microscopic polyangiitis (MPA) classically presents with rapidly progressive glomerulonephritis and sometimes alveolar haemorrhage. Systemic upset is common, together with other features such as skin lesions, GI involvement, neuropathy and pleural effusions. Patients are usually p-ANCA (myeloperoxidase) positive.

Churg–Strauss syndrome (CSS) classically presents with skin lesions (purpura or nodules), mononeuritis multiplex and peripheral eosinophilia on a background of resistant asthma. Pulmonary infiltrates and pleural or pericardial effusions due to serositis may be present. Up to 50% of patients have abdominal symptoms due to mesenteric vasculitis. Either c-ANCA or p-ANCA is present in around 40% of cases. Many CSS patients give a history of a prodromal illness characterized by allergic rhinitis, nasal polyposis and late-onset asthma that is often difficult to control.

Pathogenesis
The cause of these conditions is unclear, except in the case of PAN associated with hepatitis B infection where the disease is thought to occur as the result of an abnormal immune response to the infection.

Investigations
- Blood tests:
  - haematology: normochromic normocytic anaemia, thrombocytosis, raised ESR
  - biochemistry: raised CRP, mildly abnormal LFTs
  - immunology: c-ANCA or p-ANCA positive in about 40% of patients depending on subtype; complement C3 and C4 levels reduced in active disease.
- Biopsy:
  - renal biopsy, skin biopsy or biopsy of an affected organ can help to confirm the diagnosis.
- Imaging:
  - DEXA to assess need for osteoporosis prophylaxis.

Treatment
- Induce remission with high-dose steroids and pulse cyclophosphamide: oral prednisolone 1 mg/kg daily and

cyclophosphamide 2 mg/kg daily for 4–6 weeks or pulse methylprednisolone 10 mg/kg and cyclophosphamide 15 mg/kg every 2 weeks for up to 6 pulses

- Maintain remission with lower dose steroids and azathioprine: oral prednisolone 20 mg/24 h, reducing gradually, and azathioprine 1–2 mg/kg daily
- Co-trimoxazole (960 mg thrice weekly) as prophylaxis against *Pneumocystis* pneumonia
- PPIs (e.g. omeprazole 20 mg/24 h) as prophylaxis against stress-induced peptic ulcer
- Mesna as prophylaxis against bladder toxicity
- Antiviral therapy (in HBV-infected patients).

WEGENER'S GRANULOMATOSIS

Wegener's granulomatosis is a vasculitis that involves the upper airways and nasal passages. It presents with epistaxis, nasal crusting and sinusitis, haemoptysis, mucosal ulceration and deafness due to serous otitis media. Proptosis and diplopia may occur due to inflammation of the retro-orbital tissue. Untreated nasal disease ultimately leads to destruction of bone and cartilage. Migratory pulmonary infiltrates and nodules occur in 50% of patients and some patients present with glomerulonephritis. Patients are usually c-ANCA positive. Management is with high-dose steroids and pulse cyclophosphamide as described for PAN.

BEHÇET'S SYNDROME

Behçet's syndrome is a vasculitis that mainly targets venules. It preferentially affects some ethnic groups, including people of Turkish and Japanese descent, and is genetically associated with carriage of HLA-B51. There are a wide range of clinical features, including oral and genital ulcers, skin rash (erythema nodosum or acneiform lesions), arthralgia, migratory thrombophlebitis, uveitis, retinal vasculitis, meningitis and various focal neurological lesions. Patients with Behçet's may exhibit a pathergy reaction where a pustule develops at the site of skin trauma (e.g. intradermal skin pricking with a needle). Management is with topical steroids for oral ulceration and colchicine for skin rash and arthralgia. Thalidomide (100–300 mg/24 h for 28 days initially) can be used for resistant oral and genital ulceration. Neurological disease requires treatment with high-dose steroids and immunosuppressives.

OTHER FORMS OF VASCULITIS

Kawasaki's disease is a rare systemic vasculitis that is commonly found in Japanese children under the age of 5 years in response to an infectious trigger. *Clinical presentation* is with systemic upset (fever for more than 5 days with cervical lymphadenopathy), conjunctivitis, red lips/mouth with a 'strawberry tongue', erythema and swelling of hands and feet, skin rash, arthritis and cardiac disease (pancarditis, MI, coronary aneurysms). *Investigations* include increased platelets, WCC and CRP. *Treatment* is with high-dose i.v. gamma-globulin and aspirin.

Takayasu's arteritis is a granulomatous inflammation of the aorta and its branches. It is a rare disorder which predominantly affects young women (<50 years) with symptoms of claudication, diminished/absent pulses (arms more than legs), visual disturbance, syncope and CVA. Bruits are often heard over the carotid and subclavian vessels. *Treatment* is with steroids, cytotoxic drugs and antithrombotic agents.

Henoch–Schönlein purpura occurs in children and young adults, and generally has a good prognosis. The typical presentation is with a purpuric rash over the buttocks and lower legs, abdominal pain and an asymmetrical arthritis following an upper respiratory tract infection. Glomerulonephritis occurs in about 40% of patients and may occur up to 4 weeks after the onset of other symptoms. The diagnosis can only be confirmed by demonstrating IgA deposition within and around blood vessel walls. Corticosteroids are effective for GI and joint involvement but nephritis usually requires treatment with high-dose steroids and immunosuppressives.

CONNECTIVE TISSUE DISEASE

SYSTEMIC LUPUS ERYTHEMATOSUS

SLE is a systemic autoimmune disease which can present with a wide variety of symptoms involving several organ systems. The disease onset peaks between the 2nd and 4th decade and it is more common in women (10:1). The population prevalence is about 0.03% in Caucasians but is about 10 times higher (0.2%) in people of Afro-Caribbean descent.

Pathogenesis

The cause of SLE is unknown but autoantibody production directed against DNA and other components of the cell nucleus is a hallmark feature. This has led to the hypothesis that there may be a defect in processing apoptotic cells in SLE, leading to inappropriate display of nuclear components on the cell surface and autoantibody formation, which form immune complexes and cause vasculitis in several organ systems. Patients with inherited complement deficiency run an increased risk of developing SLE. Environmental factors such as oxidative stress, infections and UV light exposure are important trigger factors and the disease can be drug induced (hydralazine, procainamide). Genetic factors play a significant role and associations with HLA-DR2 and DR3 have been reported.

Clinical features

The clinical features of SLE are many, including:

- Polyarthritis or polyarthralgia
- Fatigue and malaise
- Photosensitive skin rash
- Focal neurological signs, psychosis, seizures, depression
- Raynaud's syndrome
- Alopecia with scarring
- Mouth ulcers
- Haemolytic anaemia, leucopenia, thrombocytopenia
- Painful oral ulceration
- Glomerulonephritis, renal failure
- Pleurisy and pericarditis, pneumonitis, pulmonary fibrosis
- Thromboembolism.

Investigations

- Blood tests:
  - haematology: haemolytic anaemia, thrombocytopenia, lymphopenia; raised ESR with active disease
  - biochemistry: CRP often normal (except during infection); abnormal U&Es in renal disease
  - immunology: positive ANA (95–99%), dsDNA (35%); RF, anticardiolipin, anti-Ro, anti-La and Sm antibodies may also be positive. Complement levels (C3 and C4) reduced during an acute flare and reduced in patients with inherited deficiency.
- Imaging:
  - periarticular osteoporosis, bone erosions usually absent
  - MRI in suspected CNS lupus.

- Urinalysis: ✗ easy test @ bedside ✗
  — proteinuria, haematuria and casts in renal disease.
- Biopsy:
  — skin biopsy for evidence of IgG and complement deposition (lupus band test)
  — renal biopsy if glomerulitis suspected.

Treatment
- Analgesics/NSAIDs for arthritis
- Intra-articular steroids for problem joints
- Hydroxychloroquine for skin and joint disease
- High-dose pulse steroids with cyclophosphamide or mycophenolate mofetil in patients with renal, cardiac or neurological involvement:
  - maintenance therapy with low-dose steroids and azathioprine
  - topical steroids for discoid lupus.

Prognosis
- Patients with mild disease have a good prognosis and the overall 10-year survival is about 85%
- Infection, renal failure and cardiovascular disease are the commonest causes of death.

SCLERODERMA

Scleroderma (or systemic sclerosis) is a connective tissue disorder affecting the skin, internal organs and vascular system which is characterized by progressive fibrosis and multiorgan failure. A more limited form of the syndrome (limited systemic sclerosis; formerly CREST syndrome) is recognized in which calcinosis, Raynaud's syndrome, oesophageal involvement, sclerodactyly and telangiectasia occur. This follows a more benign course than classic scleroderma. Disease onset is usually between the ages of 20 and 50 years and women are predominantly affected (4:1).

Pathogenesis
The pathogenesis is unknown. The disease is associated with fibroblast activation in the dermis and increased deposition of collagen, and narrowing of arterioles and small arteries associated with intimal proliferation and an inflammatory infiltrate.

Clinical presentation

- Severe Raynaud's syndrome and digital ulceration
- Skin fibrosis (sclerodactyly, microstomia)
- Telangiectasia
- Calcinosis
- Oesophageal dysmotility
- Pulmonary hypertension, pulmonary fibrosis
- Hypertension
- Renal failure
- Polyarthralgia and contractures
- Malabsorption.

Investigations

- Blood tests:
  - haematology: often normal; ESR may be raised
  - biochemistry: normal except in renal failure; CRP may be raised
  - immunology: positive ANA (90%), anti-Scl70 antibody positive (30%), anti-centromere antibody positive (80%) in limited systemic sclerosis.
- Imaging:
  - endoscopy to investigate oesophageal symptoms
  - barium studies for malabsorption
  - CXR and high-resolution CT for lung involvement.

Treatment

- Control hypertension with ACE inhibitors and other antihypertensives
- Treat oesophageal reflux and dyspepsia with PPIs and antireflux agents
- Avoid cold exposure and use vasodilators and heated gloves for Raynaud's
- Steroids and cytotoxics for pulmonary fibrosis
- Antibiotics for infected digital ulcers.

Prognosis

- 10-year survival ~60%
- Cardiovascular disease, renal failure and pulmonary hypertension are the commonest causes of death.

POLYMYOSITIS AND DERMATOMYOSITIS

These are rare diseases of unknown cause characterized by muscle weakness and inflammation. *Polymyositis* presents with proximal muscle weakness and systemic features such as fever, weight loss and fatigue. Muscle pain may also occur. Involvement of the respiratory and pharyngeal muscles may lead to aspiration pneumonia and ventilatory failure. Pulmonary fibrosis occurs in up to 30% of cases. In *dermatomyositis*, the presentation is similar but with additional features of a maculopapular rash over the extensor surfaces of the PIPJs and DIPJs and a violet discoloration of the eyelids and periorbital oedema (heliotrope rash). Investigations show a high ESR and CRP and a raised CK. Electromyography shows features of myopathy and the diagnosis is confirmed by a muscle biopsy which shows typical features of muscle fibre necrosis, regeneration and inflammatory cell infiltrate.

In many cases polymyositis or dermatomyositis occurs secondary to an occult malignancy and so it is usual to carry out routine screening for this by performing a whole body CT, GI tract imaging and mammography. Management is with high-dose steroids (prednisolone 60–80 mg/24 h). The dose is gradually reduced according to the clinical response and CK levels (which act as a marker of disease activity). Lower doses of steroids are required to maintain remission and are often combined with cytotoxic drugs such as azathioprine or methotrexate.

SJÖGREN'S SYNDROME

Sjögren's syndrome is an autoimmune disorder of unknown aetiology characterized by inflammation of the salivary and lachrymal glands. The typical age at onset is between 40 and 50 years with a female:male ratio of 9:1. The disease may be primary or occur in association with other autoimmune diseases such as RA, SLE, autoimmune thyroid disease or primary biliary cirrhosis. The typical presentation is with a dry mouth, dry 'gritty' eyes, conjunctivitis and blepharitis. Investigations show an elevated ESR and hypergammaglobulinaemia, positive ANA and RF. The Schirmer test measures tear flow over 5 mins using absorbent paper strips placed in the lower eyelid. Normally more than 6 mm of wetting occurs and this is reduced in Sjögren's syndrome. Lip biopsy is sometimes performed and reveals a lymphocytic infiltrate in the minor salivary glands. Management is symptomatic. Hypromellose eye drops are used for dry eyes. Patients with dry mouth should be advised about oral hygiene, promptly treated for infections (e.g. candidiasis) and advised to take fluids frequently.

FIBROMYALGIA

Fibromyalgia is a condition of unknown cause characterized by widespread pain affecting the muscle and soft tissues. Stressful life events are an important predisposing factor and it is often associated with depression, facial pain, IBS, sleep problems and chronic fatigue. The peak incidence is between 30 and 60 years, and it is more common in females (10:1). The overall prevalence has been estimated to be 2–4%.

Pathogenesis
The pathogenesis is unknown but neuropsychiatric factors with abnormal central processing of pain signals are thought to be involved.

Clinical presentation
- Widespread aches and pains
- Hyperalgesia with moderate digital pressure at multiple sites (Figure 5.4)
- Chronic fatigue
- Anxiety, poor concentration, depression, forgetfulness, tension headaches, IBS, paraesthesia, increased sensitivity to drug side effects.

Investigations
Haematology, biochemistry, immunology and routine imaging usually show no abnormality.

Treatment
Treatment is difficult, and essentially symptomatic in nature:

- Low-dose amitriptyline (10–25 mg at night) for pain relief; NSAIDs and analgesics are usually ineffective
- Fluoxetine for mood disturbance.

Non-pharmacological approaches include:

- Education
- Acupuncture
- Physiotherapy
- Cognitive behaviour therapy.

Prognosis
The prognosis is poor. Treatment can improve quality of life and ability to cope to an extent but is seldom curative.

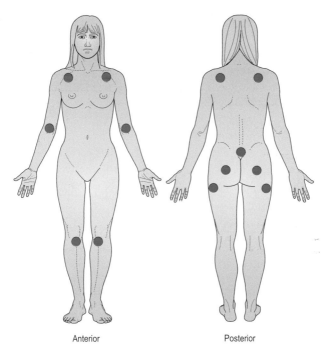

Anterior   Posterior

Figure 5.4 Regional tenderness in fibromyalgia.

CRYSTAL-INDUCED ARTHRITIS

GOUT

Gout is a form of inflammatory arthritis associated with
hyperuricaemia and deposition of uric acid crystals in the joints
and soft tissues. It most commonly presents in adults between the
ages of 20 and 40 years and is more common in men (8:1). The
population prevalence is ~0.5%.

Pathogenesis
Acute gout is caused by deposition of uric acid crystals in the
joint, which sets up an inflammatory reaction (synovitis). Patients
with gout have raised levels of uric acid in the blood due to
overproduction of uric acid or decreased excretion. Genetic
factors influence rates of uric acid production and excretion in the

normal population, and in Lesch–Nyhan syndrome there is severe overproduction of uric acid due to an enzyme defect. Increased production of uric acid also occurs in myeloproliferative and lymphoproliferative disease. Genetic factors also influence the regulation of uric acid excretion, but other important causes of reduced excretion include renal impairment, dehydration, alcohol excess and diuretics (thiazide).

Clinical presentation
- Acute gout presents with:
  — sudden onset of a painful, swollen, red, hot and tender joint
  — bursitis, tendonitis or cellulitis.
- Chronic gout presents with:
  — polyarthritis due to bone and cartilage degradation; bony ankylosis
  — soft tissue deposits of uric acid (tophi)
  — skin ulceration with extrusion of uric acid crystals.
  — Renal failure, e.g. urate nephropathy.

Investigations
- Blood tests:
  — haematology: leucocytosis and raised ESR during acute attack
  — biochemistry: raised CRP during acute attack; uric acid raised but may be normal during acute attack; abnormal U&Es in renal disease.
- Joint aspiration:
  — sterile, cloudy fluid with raised WCC and low viscosity
  — uric acid crystals may be seen under polarized light.
- Imaging:
  — punched-out bone erosions in affected joints with soft tissue swelling
  — loss of joint space, osteophytes, periarticular osteosclerosis.

Treatment
- Acute attack:
  — NSAIDs, analgesics and/or colchicines (see Chapter 8)
  — rest affected joints
  — intra-articular or systemic steroids in resistant cases.
- Long-term management:
  — reduce alcohol intake, avoid dehydration and excessive amounts of purine-rich foods (e.g. game, red meat, seafood)
  — allopurinol to reduce uric acid production (delay until after acute attack has settled)
  — probenecid or sulfinpyrazone to increase uric acid excretion.

PSEUDOGOUT

Pseudogout is an acute inflammatory arthritis associated with deposition of calcium pyrophosphate crystals in the joints. It is often associated with radiological chondrocalcinosis where calcium pyrophosphate crystals become deposited in menisci and articular cartilage. There is also a strong association with OA. It most commonly presents in adults between the ages of 60 and 80 years with a population prevalence of ~0.5%.

Pathogenesis
Pseudogout is caused by precipitation of calcium pyrophosphate crystals in the joint, which sets up an inflammatory reaction. Deposition of calcium pyrophosphate crystals in articular cartilage increases in incidence with age and affects up to 15% of people between the ages of 65 and 75 years. Genetic factors play an important role in determining susceptibility and in some cases the disease is familial and inherited in an autosomal dominant manner due to mutations in the *ANKH* gene. Chondrocalcinosis may also occur in association with other diseases including hyperparathyroidism, hypothyroidism, haemochromatosis, diabetes mellitus, Wilson's disease and acromegaly. Recognized precipitating factors for an attack include surgery, trauma, dehydration, starvation and infection.

Clinical presentation
● Sudden onset of a painful, swollen, red, hot and tender joint
● Typically affects large joints (e.g. knee, ankle, wrist).

Investigations
● Blood tests:
  — haematology: leucocytosis and raised ESR during acute attack
  — biochemistry: raised CRP during acute attack. Biochemistry may reveal evidence of predisposing disease (e.g. hypercalcaemia in primary hyperparathyroidism).
● Joint aspiration:
  — sterile, cloudy fluid with raised WCC and low viscosity
  — rhomboid-shaped CPP crystals may be seen under polarized light.
● Imaging:
  — chondrocalcinosis and changes of OA on radiograph (Figure 5.5).

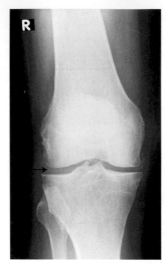

Figure 5.5 Chondrocalcinosis of the knee. This film shows calcification of the knee cartilage menisci due to crystal deposition (arrowed).

Treatment
- Acute attack:
  - — NSAIDs and analgesics
  - — rest affected joints
  - — intra-articular or systemic steroids in resistant cases.
- Long-term management:
  - — joint replacement possible if combined with OA.

OSTEOARTHRITIS

OA is the most common form of arthritis. It is characterized by cartilage damage and joint space narrowing with increased bone formation around affected joints. The hands, knees, hips and spine are most commonly affected. The incidence of OA increases markedly with age such that about 80% of people over the age of 65 have some radiological evidence of the disease. Although OA is asymptomatic in many individuals, it remains a major cause of morbidity and disability in older people.

Pathogenesis
Both genetic and environmental factors are involved in the pathogenesis of OA. A positive family history is common and

twin and family studies have shown that heritability of the disease is substantial. It is often considered to be a degenerative disease of cartilage, triggered by excessive or abnormal mechanical loading of the joint, but in many patients there is a low-grade inflammatory component, albeit intermittently. Patients with OA also tend to have high bone mass and another theory of causation is that increased density of subchondral bone causes increased biomechanical damage to articular cartilage. Recognized risk factors for OA include:

MCQ: 1st sign = cartilage swelling.

- Obesity
- Occupational damage to joints:
  — professional sportspeople
  — farmers
  — miners
- Injuries:
  — fracture affecting articular surface
  — ligament rupture
  — meniscal tear
- Coexisting disease:
  — Paget's disease of bone
  — septic arthritis
  — hypermobility
  — developmental dislocation of the hip
  — Perthes' disease.

Clinical features (Table 5.1)
The typical presentation of OA is with:

- Joint pain and stiffness, worse on movement and load bearing, typically affecting the hands, knees, hips, back and neck
- Swelling of affected joints due to osteophyte formation (Bouchard's and Heberden's nodes in the hands; Figure 5.6)
- Joint deformity (e.g. varus deformity of the knees, leg shortening)
- Crepitus, decreased range of movement and muscle wasting
- Mild synovitis and effusion
- Exacerbations and remissions
- Limp/antalgic gait.

Investigations
- Blood tests:
  — haematology and biochemistry: usually normal
  — immunology: usually normal.
- Joint aspiration:
  — sterile, viscous fluid; WCC may be slightly raised.

TABLE 5.1 Spectrum of presentations seen in osteoarthritis

Subtype	Features
Nodal OA	Nodal or primary generalized OA is less common, but has a strong genetic component which often affects women
	Nodal OA of the hands is often associated with knee and hip OA, along with the first MTP joint (hallux rigidus)
	Autoimmune complex deposition is thought to be the cause
Hip OA	Common in Caucasian populations, this category of presentation is often classified on the radiological appearance: superior-pole hip OA (common in men, unilateral, weight-bearing surfaces primarily affected) and medial cartilage loss (common in women, bilateral, coexists with nodal/hand OA)
Knee OA	Commonly presents in obese women, with a high prevalence in those ≥75 years
	Other predisposing factors are previous knee trauma, e.g. meniscal, ACL and PCL tears
	Often a bilateral condition, with OA of the medial compartment of the knee leading to a bow-leg presentation, i.e. varus deformity (cyclical deformity)
	Strong association with OA of the hand

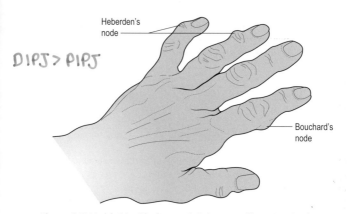

DIPJ > PIPJ

Heberden's node

Bouchard's node

Figure 5.6 Nodal OA with characteristic bony swellings. DIPJ involvement is known as Heberden's nodes and PIPJ involvement as Bouchard's nodes. Nodal OA has a propensity for the DIPJs over the PIPJs, commonly only affecting one joint at a time over a period of years. The presentation in the inflammatory phase is with pain, swelling and reduction of function in the affected hand. CMCJ and MCPJ involvement, particularly of the thumb, may coexist.

- Imaging:
  — loss of joint space, osteophytes, subchondral sclerosis and cysts on radiograph (Figure 5.7); patellofemoral OA of the knee requires a skyline view
  — cartilage erosion and bone marrow oedema in subchondral bone on MRI.
- Arthroscopy:
  — cartilage loss and erosions.

Treatment
- Analgesics/NSAIDs for pain relief (systemically or topically)
- Intra-articular steroids in patients with effusion
- Nutraceuticals:
  — glucosamine/chondroitin (evidence for benefit marginal).
- Non-pharmacological approaches:
  — education
  — weight loss
  — muscle strengthening exercises (e.g. quadriceps exercises in knee OA)
  — physiotherapy, hydrotherapy.

MCQ: hip walking stick on contralateral side.

- Surgery:
  — indicated when medical management fails to control symptoms and quality of life is impaired
  — chondrocyte transplantation (experimental stage only)
  — total knee and hip replacement (p. 139) most successful
  — realignment surgery (osteotomy) and joint fusion (arthrodesis) occasionally performed.

DISEASES OF BONE

OSTEOPOROSIS

Osteoporosis is a common disease that increases in incidence with age. It affects women more often than men and is characterized by low BMD, increased bone fragility and an increased risk of fracture. Osteoporosis is defined to exist when BMD values are reduced by more than 2.5 standard deviations (T-score units) below the value observed in young healthy adults (see Chapter 3). The prevalence of osteoporosis increases with age and fractures related to osteoporosis are estimated to affect 30% of women and 12% of men at some time in life. The cost of treating osteoporotic fractures in the UK is about £1.2 million and most of this is

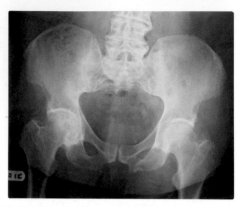

Figure 5.7 OA of the hip. Changes include joint space narrowing due to loss of cartilage, subarticular sclerosis, subchondral cysts and osteophyte formation causing 'lipping' at joint margins. Pathological features of OA are subchondral cysts, bursitis, periarticular osteophytes, subchondral sclerosis, fibrillation and loss of cartilage, and synovial hyperplasia.

accounted for by hip fractures, which cause substantial morbidity and are associated with significant mortality.

Pathogenesis
The main cause of osteoporosis is increased bone loss associated with age and postmenopausal oestrogen deficiency. Both factors cause uncoupling of bone resorption from bone formation such that the amount of bone removed by osteoclasts (bone-resorbing cells) during remodelling of bone is not matched by the amount replaced by osteoblasts (bone-forming cells). Ageing itself also plays a key role in the pathogenesis of osteoporotic fractures since the risk of falling is increased due to various factors such as poor vision, muscle weakness and postural instability. The most important risk factors include:

- Family history
- Early menopause
- Low body weight
- Poor diet
- Drug treatment: corticosteroids, aromatase inhibitors, GnRH therapy
- Coexisting disease:
  — chronic inflammatory diseases
  — malabsorption
  — hypogonadism.   *hyperthyroidism*

Clinical features

The clinical presentation of osteoporosis is with <u>fractures</u>. These can affect any bone, but the three most common sites are the <u>wrist, hip and spine.</u> A previous fracture is associated with a greatly increased risk of future fractures. Clinical signs of osteoporosis are restricted to patients with fracture and include:

● Height loss and kyphosis (vertebral fracture)
● Painful, shortened externally rotated hip (hip fracture)
● Pain and deformity of affected bone (other fractures).

Investigations

● Blood tests:
 — haematology: normal in idiopathic osteoporosis; raised ESR in inflammatory disease or in osteoporosis secondary to myeloma
 — biochemistry: normal in idiopathic osteoporosis; abnormalities may be detected in secondary osteoporosis (e.g. hypercalcaemia, hyperparathyroidism, abnormal thyroid function tests in thyrotoxicosis).
● Imaging:
 — radiographs may show evidence of fracture or osteopenia
 — DEXA scans show reduced BMD (see Chapter 3).

Treatment (Table 5.2; see Chapter 8)

● <u>Bisphosphonates</u> to inhibit bone resorption:
 — alendronic acid (alendronate), risedronate, ibandronic acid (ibandronate) orally
 — zoledronic acid (zoledronate) and ibandronic acid (ibandronate) intravenously.
● Calcium and vitamin D supplements
● Other anti-osteoporosis treatments include:
 — calcitonin, raloxifene, strontium ranelate, HRT
 — parathyroid hormone – used in severe osteoporosis.

TABLE 5.2 Thresholds for initiation of drug treatment of osteoporosis	
Patient group	*Treatment threshold (T-score)*
Postmenopausal osteoporosis	−2.5
Osteoporosis in men	−2.5
Corticosteroid-induced osteoporosis	−1.5

OSTEOMALACIA

Osteomalacia is a disease characterized by reduced mineralization of bone, which in most cases is due to vitamin D deficiency. When osteomalacia occurs in the growing skeleton it is known as rickets. Muslim women and elderly housebound individuals are at increased risk of osteomalacia, since vitamin D is mostly derived from exposure to sunlight.

Pathogenesis

Osteomalacia and rickets occur because of deficiency of the active metabolite of vitamin D (1,25(OH)2D), which is necessary for efficient absorption of calcium and phosphate from the intestine. The most common cause is deficiency of the precursor cholecalciferol, which is synthesized in the skin from 7-dehydrocholesterol under the influence of UV light or obtained from the diet. Cholecalciferol is converted by the liver to 25(OH)D and then by the kidneys to (1,25(OH)2D), which is biologically active. When vitamin deficiency occurs, intestinal calcium absorption is low, stimulating production of parathyroid hormone, which causes removal of calcium and phosphate from the bone, resulting in poor mineralization. Less common causes of osteomalacia and rickets include:

- Inherited metabolic defects in vitamin D metabolism (vitamin D resistant rickets)
- Inherited defects in phosphate metabolism (hypophosphataemic rickets)
- Acquired defects in phosphate metabolism (tumour-induced osteomalacia)
- Chronic renal failure (failure of 1,25(OH)2D synthesis)
- Bisphosphonates, aluminium toxicity.

Clinical presentation

The classic presenting features of osteomalacia include:

- Bone pain and/or tenderness
- Muscle weakness and fatigue
- General malaise
- Fracture.

The presenting features of rickets include:

- Bone pain and deformity
- Bone expansion at the epiphyseal plate

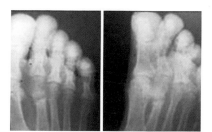

Figure 5.8 A pseudofracture of the 2nd metatarsal due to osteomalacia. Other changes in adults include widespread density changes due to cortical bone loss. A low-density narrow strip caused by stressed repair of a fracture on the compression side may be seen; this is known as a 'Looser's zone'.

- Delayed development and failure to thrive
- Tetany and seizures.

Investigations

- Blood tests:
  — haematology: normal
  — biochemistry: low calcium and phosphate; raised ALP, raised PTH, low 25(OH)D.
- Imaging:
  — radiographs show widening of the epiphyses in rickets, osteopenia and fractures or pseudofractures (Figure 5.8) in adults.
- Bone biopsy:
  — shows increased thickness and extent of osteoid seams (uncalcified bone matrix).

Treatment

- Ergocalciferol 10 000 U/24 h, plus calcium supplements in vitamin D deficient rickets
- Active vitamin D metabolites in rickets associated with chronic renal failure and in vitamin D resistant rickets
- Phosphate supplements plus active vitamin D metabolites in hypophosphataemic rickets: monitor serum ALP levels during treatment (values normalize when healing occurs).

PAGET'S DISEASE

Paget's is a common bone disease characterized by focal increases in bone remodelling, which result in the production of abnormal bone that is mechanically weak. The bones most commonly affected include the pelvis, spine, skull, femur and tibia. Paget's disease is uncommon under the age of 50 but the prevalence doubles each decade thereafter to affect about 8% of the UK population over the age of 80. Men and women are affected equally. There are marked ethnic differences in susceptibility. The disease is common in the UK and other parts of Europe (except Scandinavia), but is extremely rare in the Far East and the Indian subcontinent.

Pathogenesis
Genetic factors play an important role and mutations in the *SQSTM1* gene are found in about 40–50% of patients with a positive family history of the disease. These mutations lead to increased osteoclast activity. Environmental factors also contribute and suggested triggers for the disease include a poor diet, exposure to infections and skeletal damage or repetitive mechanical loading.

Clinical presentation
Paget's disease is often asymptomatic but typical presenting features include:

- Bone pain
- Bone expansion and deformity
- Pathological fracture (Figure 5.9)
- Increased temperature over an affected bone
- Hearing loss.

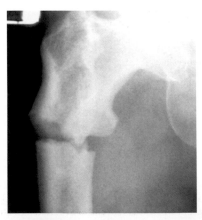

Figure 5.9 Pathological fractures are often seen with Paget's disease.

Less common features include:

- Hypercalcaemia (with immobilization)
- High output cardiac failure (increased blood flow through bone)
- Spinal cord compression/spinal stenosis
- Hydrocephalus
- Osteosarcoma.

Investigations
- Blood tests:
  — haematology: normal
  — biochemistry: raised ALP with otherwise normal biochemistry.
- Imaging:
  — radiographs show bone expansion and deformity with areas of osteosclerosis alternating with areas of osteolysis
  — MRI for suspected spinal stenosis and cord compression.
- Bone biopsy:
  — seldom required for diagnosis, but shows markedly increased bone turnover, marrow fibrosis, giant osteoclasts and woven bone.

Treatment
Main indication is bone pain.

- Antiresorptive drugs to reduce bone turnover: (bisphosphonates)
  — risedronate, tiludronic acid (tiludronate), etidronate orally
  — pamidronate, zoledronic acid (zoledronate) intravenously
  — serum ALP is a marker for suppression of bone turnover.
- Analgesics/NSAIDs for pain control.
- Surgery:
  — fracture fixation
  — joint replacement (secondary OA)
  — spinal stenosis
  — osteotomy for deformity
  — osteosarcoma (prognosis poor even with amputation).

REFLEX SYMPATHETIC DYSTROPHY SYNDROME

Also known as Sudeck's atrophy or algodystrophy, this syndrome is characterized by bone pain, swelling of the affected limb and localized osteoporosis. It is thought to be due to a disturbance in neurovascular function, and often follows an episode of trauma.

Clinical presentation
- Persistent pain beyond the specific site of injury
- Feeling of burning (causalgia)
- Primarily there is heat, erythema and swelling of the affected area
- Stiff and tender joints (varying degrees) with a decreased ROM
- Secondary hypersensitivity/hyperreflexia and autonomic disturbance with skin atrophy and pallor.

Treatment
- Lifestyle factors:
  — education
  — physiotherapy.
- Analgesia (see Chapter 8):
  — NSAIDs
  — calcitonin, bisphosphonates, bretylium (postganglionic sympathetic blocker), amitriptyline.

CHAPTER 6

PAEDIATRIC ORTHOPAEDICS AND RHEUMATOLOGY

BONE STRUCTURE AND INJURY

STRUCTURE OF YOUNG BONE

The structure of bone differs when growing. Normal bone comprises the metaphysis, diaphysis and epiphysis. In growing bone, the epiphyseal plates have not fused (Figure 6.1) and thus injury to growing bone is classified differently. In addition, trauma to growing bone can lead to complications in later life, such as deformity and growth disturbance. However, children's bones do heal more rapidly than those of adults, thus prompt and effective management often produces good results.

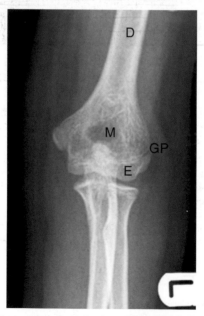

Figure 6.1 The anatomy of growing bone. The fusion of growth plates at the elbow are of particular importance. In ascending order of when they occur: capitulum (1 year old), radial head (3 years old), medial epicondyle (6 years old), trochlea and olecranon (8 years old), lateral epicondyle (12 years old). D, diaphysis; E, epiphysis; GP, growth plate, M, metaphysis.

→ CRMTOL

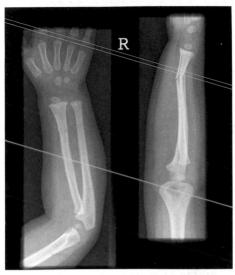

Figure 6.2 Greenstick fracture of the distal radius and ulna.

FRACTURE TYPES IN CHILDREN

The fracture classification system laid out in Chapter 7 can also be used for children. However, some fracture types are more common in children. These include:

- Greenstick fracture (Figure 6.2): a fracture where the bone bends as it does not fracture completely across, i.e. one side of the cortex often remains intact. Angulation and instability of the fracture are possible
- Buckle fracture (Figure 6.3): a fracture where the bone buckles but no fracture line is seen, i.e. the cortex often remains intact. Angulation and instability of the fracture are uncommon.

SALTER–HARRIS INJURY CLASSIFICATION

Five patterns of injury involving the growth plate in children are described in the Salter–Harris classification (Figure 6.4):

1. A transverse fracture with complete displacement along the epiphyseal plate line only (commonly seen in scurvy). Growth disturbance is rare

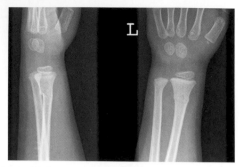

Figure 6.3 Buckle fracture of the distal radius.

2. Epiphysis detachment due to fracture, with an attached metaphysis fragment. This is the commonest type of fracture
3. A displaced epiphyseal fracture fragment. The fracture may be intra-articular. Can lead to growth disturbance
4. A fracture line that is consistent through the epiphysis, epiphyseal plate and metaphysis. The fracture may be intra-articular. The epiphyseal plate is very susceptible to growth disturbance due to early growth plate fusion
5. Compression injury leading to obliteration of the epiphyseal growth plate. Fracture type most commonly associated with growth arrest and deformity, e.g. shortening of the affected limb.

A sixth pattern of fracture has been described, since production of the original classification, as part of the new Peterson classification. This fracture, often open, leads to detachment of a section of the epiphysis, epiphyseal plate and metaphysis (Figure 6.4). The epiphyseal plate is very susceptible to growth disturbance due to early growth plate fusion and often requires primary surgical management.

INJURIES IN CHILDREN[1]

Supracondylar fractures

Supracondylar fractures are common in children, particularly boys, following a direct fall onto the elbow or a fall onto an extended (outstretched) hand. *Clinical presentation* is with elbow

[1] Always be aware of non-accidental injury in children.

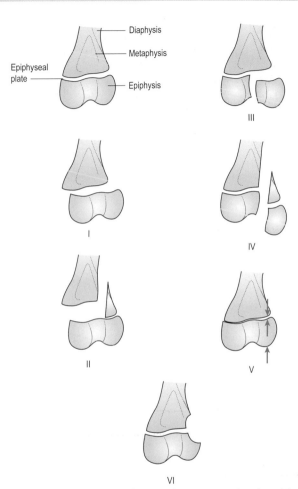

Figure 6.4 Salter–Harris classification of injury that involves the epiphyseal plate. Fractures involving the plate commonly occur in the hypertrophic region of the plate. The new Peterson classification adds a type VI fracture to the original Salter–Harris classification.

pain, tenderness and swelling, with posterior displacement of the distal fragment common. It is essential to determine the neurovascular status of the affected limb (radial and brachial pulse, capillary refill time, median nerve sensation distribution). *Investigations* include AP and lateral X-rays of the injured elbow

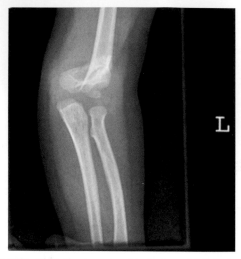

Figure 6.5 Grossly displaced supracondylar fracture of the elbow.

(Figure 6.5) from which the degree and direction of displacement can be determined (Baumann's angle – the angle subtended by a line through the growth plate of the capitulum with a line through the long axis of the humerus). *Treatment* is dependent on the degree of displacement. Fractures with minimal displacement can be treated with immobilization in an above-elbow backslab (elbow at 90°) and sling. Fractures with significant displacement can be treated with reduction under general anaesthesia, followed by fixation with K-wires for unstable or irreducible fractures. Once again, it is essential to determine the neurovascular status of the affected limb post reduction, as well as performing a post-reduction radiograph. *Complications* include malunion, compartment syndrome, soft tissue injury (brachial artery and major nerves), heterotopic ossification (stiffness) and long-term deformity (e.g. cubitus varus).

Condylar fractures

Medial and lateral condyle fractures are relatively uncommon in children. *Clinical presentation* is with elbow pain, tenderness and swelling, with lateralization to the affected side. It is essential to determine the neurovascular status of the affected limb (radial

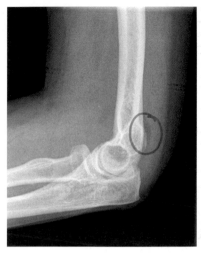

Figure 6.6 An elevated fad pad may be a useful sign to determine elbow pathology when no actual fracture is seen. It is also useful to look for the position of the anterior humeral line as it may be displaced in supracondylar fractures. A displaced radiocapitular line is indicative of an elbow or radial head dislocation.

↗ medial condyle

and brachial pulse, capillary refill time, ulnar nerve sensation distribution). *Investigations* include AP and lateral views of the injured elbow, which may only show an elevated fat pad (Figure 6.6). *Treatment* is dependent on the degree of displacement. Fractures with no displacement can be treated with immobilization in an above-elbow splint. Fractures with displacement can be treated with reduction (closed or open), with or without internal fixation. *Complications* include mal- or non-union, soft tissue injury (ulnar nerve in medial condyle fractures), recurrent dislocation and long-term deformity.

Pulled elbow
A pulled elbow is common following a 'yank' on a child's wrist leading to subluxation of the radial head out of the annular ligament (some suggest it is a dislocation of the proximal radioulnar joint). *Clinical presentation* is with elbow pain and forced extension. *Investigations* are only required when the diagnosis is in doubt. *Treatment* is with immediate reduction.

G "sweet" test

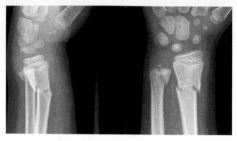

Figure 6.7 A distal radial fracture with ~30° dorsal angulation. There is a Salter–Harris type IV fracture of the distal ulna.

Distal forearm fractures   *eg. Colles'*

Distal forearm fractures are the most common site of injury in children, with the buckle, greenstick and Salter–Harris (type II) fracture types commonly seen in this region. Distal radial fractures often occur following a fall onto an extended (outstretched) hand. *Clinical presentation* is with wrist pain, tenderness and swelling, with posterior displacement of the distal fragment common in complete fracture. Gross deformity may be apparent. It is again good practice to determine the neurovascular status of the affected limb. *Investigations* include AP and lateral views of the injured wrist (Figure 6.7). *Treatment* is dependent on the type of fracture and the degree of displacement (Table 6.1). Reduction is via MUA, with immobilization using an above-elbow POP. *Complications* are uncommon but include malunion, non-union, compartment syndrome and deformity.

FOOSH

DISORDERS OF THE HIP

DIFFERENTIAL DIAGNOSIS OF A CHILDHOOD LIMP

See Table 6.2.

DEVELOPMENTAL DYSPLASIA OF THE HIP (DDH)

This congenital abnormality is relatively common. At birth the incidence of hip instability is 5–20/1000, whilst at 3 weeks this number has dropped to 1.5/1000 due to natural stabilization of

TABLE 6.1 Treatment options for distal radial fractures in children.*

Fracture type	Treatment options
Buckle	Immobilization with tubigrip or rarely plaster
Greenstick	(Other factors, including remodelling potential and age, need to be considered when determining optimal treatment. Angle is debatable.)
<15° angulation	Immobilization with plaster
>15° angulation	Reduction followed by immobilization with plaster (X-ray check 1 week)
Salter–Harris	
Stable post reduction	Reduction followed by immobilization with plaster
Unstable post reduction	Fixation, e.g. with K-wires (rare)
Complete	
Stable post reduction	Reduction followed by immobilization with plaster (X-ray check 1 week)
Unstable post reduction	Fixation, e.g. with K-wires

*Rotational disruption requires active treatment.

TABLE 6.2 The common diagnoses for a child presenting with a limp, categorized by site and age

Site	Diagnosis	Usual age range
General	Osteomyelitis Septic arthritis Connective tissue disease Trauma Tumour	Any
Spine	Discitis	3 months to 8 years
Hip	DDH	Infancy, but >1 year if delayed
	Perthes' disease	3–11 years
	Transient synovitis	4–9 years
	Slipped upper femoral epiphysis	10–16 years

the hip joint during this period. It is more common in girls (6–8:1), the left hip (4:1), and occurs bilaterally in 10–30% of cases.

DDH occurs where the femoral head does not sit consistently in a shallow and sharply slanting acetabulum, causing the joint capsule to be stretched and the ligaments lax. The femoral head moves out of position superiorly and posteriorly (Figure 6.8),

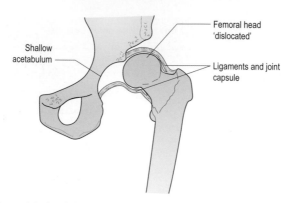

Figure 6.8 The abnormal positioning of the developing femoral head relative to the shallow acetabulum. Potential hereditary features of DDH include acetabular dysplasia and joint laxity.

leading to the impeded development of both the shallow acetabulum and proximal femur (head and neck). DDH includes a spectrum of abnormalities:

- Shallow acetabulum with dysplasia (hip in joint but dislocatable)
- Neonatal dislocation (reducible)
- Neonatal dislocation (irreducible, possibly because the labrum, lax joint capsule and/or epiphyseal plate are obstructing reduction)
- Frank subluxation/dislocation in an older child (reducible, irreducible).

Risk factors
- Genetic:
  — increased probability in girls and if a relative has DDH, i.e. a family history of DDH
  — concomitant congenital deformities, e.g. plagiocephaly, torticollis, club foot, spinal deformity (neural tube defects), scoliosis, Down's syndrome, metatarsus adductus.
- Perinatal:
  — breech birth, large babies, oligohydramnios, multiple births, e.g. twins, premature, C-section, first-born
  — poor postnatal care
  — older mothers.
- Ethnicity:
  — seen in populations, e.g. Eskimos of North America.

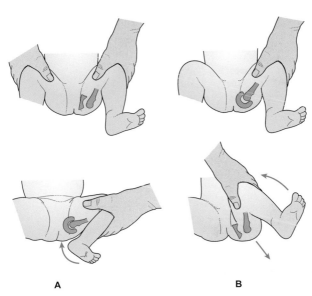

Figure 6.9 (A) Ortolani's test. (B) Barlow's test.

Clinical presentation (early)
Examination of *all* babies should occur when born, and at
6 weeks, for hip instability. Two tests that are commonly
performed are described below.

● Ortolani's test (Figure 6.9A):
   — supine, hips and knees bilaterally flexed to 90°
   — place fingers over greater trochanters, with thumbs over
     inner thigh
   — gently abduct both hips
   — negative (normal) = complete and unimpeded 90° of hip
     abduction
   — positive (DDH) = impeded abduction with a palpable and
     audible jerk as the femoral head *reduces* and enters the
     acetabulum, followed by full unimpeded hip abduction.
● Barlow's test (Figure 6.9B):
   — supine, hips flexed to 90° and adducted
   — stabilize pelvis with thumbs in the groin
   — gently push the thighs posteriorly towards the couch
   — negative (normal) = no dislocation of femoral head achieved

— positive (DDH) = femoral head slips over the posterior lip and out of the acetabulum and back in again, i.e. the hip is unstable and *dislocating*.

Clinical presentation (late)

Examination of babies at 6-month intervals during the first 2 years of life may identify late signs.

- Unilateral DDH:
  — limited abduction of affected hip
  — asymmetrical skin contours over thigh
  — delayed walking
  — Trendelenburg gait due to a dysplastic hip giving a shortened leg with partial external rotation of the leg.
- Bilateral DDH:
  — fewer features
  — impeded abduction at both hip joints
  — broadened perineal space.

Investigations

- Ultrasound:
  — early investigation (<25 weeks of age)
  — determines the characteristics of the acetabulum, as well as the relative location of the femoral head
  — potential screening tool.
- Hip (AP and lateral) and pelvic radiographs:
  — late investigation (as awaiting capital femoral epiphyses ossification)
  — may show a shallow acetabulum with a dislocated and immature femoral head
  — use Shenton's, Hilgenreiner's and Perkin's lines.

Treatment (Table 6.3)

Diagnosis and treatment at birth give the best prognosis, with follow-up surveillance necessary for all confirmed, treated or at-risk cases. Treatment options depend on the timing and severity of presentation. They include:

- Immobilization with an abduction splint:
  — confirm reduction of femoral head within acetabulum
  — Pavlik harness or von Rosen splint
  — steer clear of position extremes as there is a risk of avascular necrosis of the femoral head (Figure 6.10).
- Slow closed reduction via persistent traction:
  — hips are held in 60° flexion, 40° abduction and 20° medial rotation, firstly in plaster, and later perhaps in a splint.

TABLE 6.3 Treatment options at the various stages of DDH*

Timing	Treatment options
Early (<6 months)	Multiple nappies and reassessment with ultrasound within 3–6 weeks Moderate abduction splint with the hips flexed at 100°, e.g. Pavlik harness
Delayed (<6 years)	Gradual persistent traction then closed reduction and splintage Gradual persistent traction then open reduction ± femoral or pelvic osteotomy
Late (>6 years)	Open reduction ± femoral or pelvic osteotomy None Delayed hip arthroplasty or arthrodesis

*Imaging (ultrasound, radiograph or arthrogram) is required at all stages of treatment to confirm reduction and acetabular development. Treatment for bilateral DDH, or patients who present after 10 years of age, is often for severe pain and/or deformity.

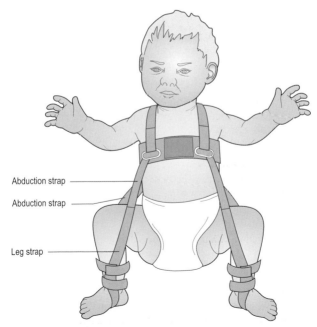

Abduction strap

Abduction strap

Leg strap

Figure 6.10 Pavlik harness used in the early treatment of DDH.

- Open reduction ± femoral varus derotation or pelvic osteotomy
- Hip arthroplasty or arthrodesis.

Complications
- The complications of frank dislocation are poor (false) development of the acetabulum and femoral epiphysis, with subsequent secondary OA and osteonecrosis possible.

PERTHES' DISEASE

Legg–Calvé–Perthes' is an idiopathic osteonecrosis of the capital femoral epiphysis (femoral head). The incidence is ~1 in 12000 and peaks between the ages of 4 and 8 years, but is seen between 3 and 11 years. It is more common in boys (4 : 1) and occurs bilaterally in 10–20% of cases. A better prognosis is seen with younger patients.

The primary blood supply to the femoral head in early childhood (3–7 years) is the vulnerable lateral epiphyseal vessels of the retinacula. Osteonecrosis in Perthes' is most likely due to the stretching and tamponade of these vessels as a result of an effusion due to injury or synovial inflammation causing prolonged ischaemic episodes and partial necrosis of the femoral head. The speed of the subsequent revascularization and healing of the necrotic zone, along with the size of epiphysis damaged, determines whether the reossification and growth process that eventually occurs produces a deformed femoral head that will cause problems with it fitting within the acetabulum.

Risk factors
- Genetic, e.g. family history of Perthes'
- Perinatal (small babies).

Clinical presentation
- Hip and/or knee pain with an associated limp
- Hip movements normal apart from reduced abduction and internal rotation.

Investigations
Four classification systems, based on radiological appearance, are commonly used to grade disease severity or determine outcome. They are:

- Catterall: quantity of femoral head affected, four grades
- Salter–Thompson: length of subchondral fracture line, two grades

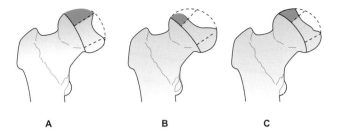

Ⓐ Grade A: normal pillar height
Ⓑ Grade B: >50% height maintained
Ⓒ Grade C: <50% height maintained

Figure 6.11 The Herring (lateral pillar) classification is arguably the most effective grading system for the assessment of unilateral Perthes' disease.

- Herring (Figure 6.11): loss of lateral femoral head height, three grades
- Stulberg: congruency of femoral head with acetabulum, five grades.

The recommended investigations are:

- Hip (AP and lateral) and pelvic radiographs (Figure 6.12):
  — early changes: ↑ articular space; ↑ density and ↓ size of femoral head epiphysis; crescent sign (sub-chondral)
  — late changes: fragmentation, fissuring, displacement, collapse and/or fracture of the femoral head epiphysis with subsequent deformity and remodelling; joint subluxation; rarefaction (Gage's sign).
- MRI or bone scan may be necessary.

Treatment
Treatment options depend on the severity of the disease.

- Mild to moderate disease:
  — bed rest (no weight bearing) with traction until pain free (~4 weeks)
  — physiotherapy
  — follow-up with imaging is essential.
- Moderate to severe disease:
  — maintained reduction of the femoral head, contained within the acetabulum using an abduction frame, plaster or splint

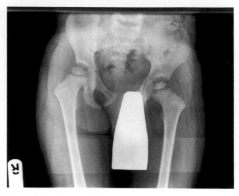

Figure 6.12 Perthes' disease of the left hip. The left femoral epiphysis is flattened, irregular and mildly sclerotic. Metaphyseal and epiphyseal rarefaction are severe signs.

   — surgery with osteotomy (usually varus) of the femur and/or
      pelvis is an alternative
   — outcome is best when performed at an early age.
● In severe cases with a very deformed femoral head and
  acetabulum that are not 'congruent' (do not match each other),
  the prognosis is poor and total hip replacement may be
  necessary at a later date.

Complications
● Pain and loss of function
● Deformities, e.g. limb shortening (severe deformity can be a
  cause of early-onset OA)
● Osteochondritis dissecans (capital femoral epiphysis).

SLIPPED UPPER FEMORAL EPIPHYSIS (SUFE)

SUFE is characterized by a posterior–inferior displacement of the
upper femoral epiphysis due to a fracture at the growth plate (a
form of pathological type I Salter–Harris growth plate fracture).
This is possibly due to a fault at the plate, e.g. poor cartilage
growth, or to an excess of forces running through it, e.g. an
overweight child.

   The disorder is very uncommon and peaks in the pubescent
years (10–16 years). It is more common in boys (3 : 1) and occurs
bilaterally in ~25% of cases, of which ~25% occur at the same

time. It is possibly associated with a disorder of growth and gonadal hormone as many patients affected are/have:

- Obese (~60%)
- Tall
- Late sexual development.

Clinical presentation
- History of injury in about one-third of presentations
- Pain (groin, hip and/or knee)
- Limp
- Decreased range of movement, in particular flexion, abduction and internal rotation
- Limb lies in external rotation and may be shortened.

Investigations
- Hip (AP and frog lateral) and pelvic radiographs:
  — look for displacement of the head (Trethowan's sign is present if a line along the lateral edge of the femoral neck does not continue to include any portion of the upper femoral epiphysis).

Treatment
- Mild displacement:
  — screw or pin fixation in given position.
- Moderate displacement:
  — pin
  — femoral neck osteotomy for deformity (if needed).
- Severe displacement:
  — possibly primary femoral neck osteotomy.

Complications
- Avascular necrosis of the femoral head, particularly if reduction is attempted
- Malunion, cartilage breakdown and avascular necrosis leading to secondary OA
- Contralateral slip (prophylactic fixation may be necessary)
- Coxa vara due to malunion.

TRANSIENT SYNOVITIS OF THE HIP

Otherwise known as irritable hip, transient synovitis of the hip is a self-limiting hypertrophic inflammatory disorder of the hip joint. No cause has been identified as definitive. However, the following are thought to be related:

● History of injury
● Recent viral infection, e.g. URTI
● Allergy.

The disorder is very common and peaks in the prepubescent years (3–10 years). It is more common in boys (2:1).

Clinical presentation
● History of pre-dated infection or injury in some cases
● Pain (groin, hip and/or knee)
● Limp
● Decreased range of movement (mild)
● Involuntary muscle spasm
● Systemic upset, e.g. fever.

Investigations
● Blood tests:
   — mildly raised ESR and WCC. If these markers, as well as CRP, are significantly raised, a diagnosis of sepsis must be considered.
● Hip (AP and lateral) and pelvic radiographs:
   — often normal
   — exclude other causes.
● Ultrasound:
   — demonstrates effusion
   — often requested in conjunction with a planned joint aspiration. It is important to exclude septic arthritis so samples should be sent to microbiology for Gram stain and culture.

Treatment
● Bed rest (~1 week) and analgesia
● Traction if necessary
● Physiotherapy and massage
● Advise should improve within 2–3 weeks.

DISORDERS OF THE KNEE

Patellar instability is discussed in Chapter 4.

OSTEOCHONDRITIS DISSECANS

Osteochondritis dissecans can occur at any joint, but is commonly seen in children's knees. It is characterized by damage to a region of the maturing epiphysis in susceptible children, especially the medial femoral condyle. A compression injury here is likely to be secondary to trauma, e.g. stress or traction, leading to inflammation, ischaemia and possibly avascular necrosis of the affected epiphysis. In children, the fragment rarely detaches, and healing is the norm. High-dose steroids are a risk factor.

Two other specific types of osteochondritis dissecans (traction apophysitis) found in the knee are:

- **Osgood–Schlatter disease**: tibial tuberosity
- **Sinding-Larsen–Johansson syndrome**: apex of patella.

Clinical presentation
- Pain in the knee:
  — may be localized to affected bone, e.g. over the tibial tuberosity
  — sporadic
  — worse at maximal extension and flexion, but with full range of movement.
- Swelling, effusion or locking of the joint
- Limp.

Investigations
- Knee (AP and lateral) radiographs:
  — loose bodies
  — area of high density (sclerosis)
  — osseous fragmentation.
- CT or MRI if necessary.

Treatment
- Analgesia
- Physiotherapy, rest and/or immobilization
- Surgery:
  — pinning or removal of displaced bone fragment.

DISORDERS OF THE FOOT

CLUB FOOT (CONGENITAL TALIPES EQUINOVARUS)

Neonatal club foot is due to atrophy and growth failure of the calf and medial soft tissues (e.g. joint capsule, tibialis posterior) leading to a characteristic deformity of the foot:

- Equinus is the foot pointing downwards due to the hindfoot being forced up because of a taut Achilles tendon (plantarflexion)
- Adduction and supination of the fore-foot relative to the hindfoot
- Total hindfoot inversion with direction towards the midline (varus position).

This disorder has an incidence of 1–2/1000 births, with higher figures seen in the developing world. It is more common in boys (2–3 : 1), the right foot and occurs bilaterally in 30–50% of cases. Recurrence is not uncommon, possibly requiring further surgery.

Risk factors
- Genetic:
  — increased probability if a relative is affected, i.e. a family history of club foot
  — concomitant congenital deformities, e.g. DDH, spina bifida, myelomeningocoele, Down's syndrome.
- Perinatal:
  — maternal alcohol, smoking and/or i.v. drug use.

Clinical presentation
- Apparent at birth
- Decreased range of movement with passive foot eversion and dorsiflexion limited
- Calf muscles wasting
- Leg shortening due to shortening of the tibia.

Investigations
- Prenatal scan (20 weeks):
  — diagnosis can sometimes be made at this stage of fetal development although false-positive 'diagnoses' are frequent.
- Foot radiographs (bilateral AP and dorsiflexion lateral):
  — altered positioning of the talus relative to the calcaneum
  — subluxation of the talonavicular joint.

There are many classification systems that can be used to grade disease severity and/or determine treatment and outcome. Those commonly employed are Pirani, Harold–Walker, Goldner and Dimeglio.

Treatment (Table 6.4)
Treatment options depend on the timing of presentation and response to treatment, but none is cosmetically definitive. They include:

TABLE 6.4 Treatment options at the various stages of congenital talipes equinovarus

Timing	Treatment options
<3 months	Ponseti method Regular manipulations of the affected foot/feet Maintain repositioning with splint or plaster
>3 months	Release of the posterior compartment and lengthening of the muscles and tendons Maintain correction with K-wires and splint
Delayed	Release and removal of soft tissue and bone, respectively Triple arthrodesis in adulthood and in children >10 years

- Conservative (the Ponseti method is a popular modern method of treatment which is mainly non-operative):
  — physiotherapy
  — immobilization in the correct position using plastering or strapping.
- Surgical:
  — posterior release with lengthening of the medial soft tissues followed by postoperative immobilization (e.g. Denis Browne splint)
  — release and removal of soft tissue and bone, respectively
  — triple arthrodesis (fusion of subtalar, talonavicular and calcaneocuboid) in adulthood for delayed presentation or recurrence.

Complications

If the abnormality is not corrected early enough, growth leads to permanent and abnormal secondary bone changes, in particular damage to the talonavicular joint due to medial subluxation of the navicular bone. Post-treatment complications include:

- Pain, stiffness and muscle weakness
- Avascular necrosis of the talus
- Recurrence and/or deformity.

JUVENILE IDIOPATHIC ARTHRITIS

Juvenile idiopathic arthritis (JIA) is a continuing (≥6 weeks) inflammatory arthritis, which commences before the age of 16 years, in the absence of an identifiable cause (e.g. sepsis).

TABLE 6.5 JIA subtypes, presentations and prognosis

Subtype	Presentation	Prognosis (Complications)
Oligoarthritis (50%)	1–4 joints affected within 6 months Young girls (~3 years) Positive ANA and/or HLA-DR5 (50%) Asymmetrical in the lower limbs (knees and ankles) No systemic disturbance and RF negative	(Uveitis)
Persisting	25–30% of these patients	Good to excellent
Extending	Progressive polyarthritis after 6 months	Poor
Polyarthritis (35%) RF negative (90%)	5 or more joints affected within 6 months Young girls, symmetrical, any joint in all four limbs Cervical spine (result in surgical cervical fusion) TMJ (poorly matured mandible and receding chin)	Poor
RF positive (10%)	Older girls (>8 years) Similar course to RA (e.g. hands, wrists) Erosions, joint destruction, nodules, systemic effects Association with HLA-DR4	Adulthood (~60%)
Systemic arthritis (10%)	Arthritis with fever for >2 weeks (Still's disease) Young girls and boys Intermittent pyrexia (>2 weeks) with a maculopapular rash, arthritis, lymphadenopathy, myalgia, hepatosplenomegaly, pericarditis, anaemia, pleurisy Raised inflammatory markers and a thrombocytosis	Recurrence common (Chronic polyarthritis, secondary amyloidosis)
Other (5%) Psoriatic arthritis	Arthritis (few joints but destructive) + psoriasis, or Arthritis + family history of psoriasis + nail pitting or dactylitis Form seen in children is similar to that found in adults	Moderate (Uveitis)
Enthesitis arthritis	Older boys, asymmetrical in the lower limb Arthritis + enthesitis or arthritis +2 of associated features: sacroiliitis, HLA-B27 (75%), anterior uveitis and a family history of spondyloarthritis, uveitis or IBD	Moderate (Ankylosing spondylitis)

TMJ, temporomandibular joint.

This disorder is relatively uncommon, with an incidence of 20–80/100 000. It affects boys and girls equally.

The cause of the disease is unknown, but – like adult RA – both hereditary and environmental factors are likely to be important in triggering an autoimmune response. RF is usually negative.

JIA is classified in relation to the pattern of disease. Pauciarticular (or oligoarticular) disease is the most common, followed by polyarticular disease. A few patients present with polyarticular disease in association with systemic features such as rash, fever, hepatosplenomegaly and anaemia (**Still's disease**). Very rarely, psoriatic arthritis and ankylosing spondylitis present in children. Details of the different disease subtypes (as defined by the International League against Rheumatism), their presentation and prognosis are shown in Table 6.5.

Treatment
- Physiotherapy and hydrotherapy:
  — improve power and range of movements in affected joints.
- NSAIDs:
  — avoid aspirin due to risk of Reye's syndrome.
- Long-term steroids:
  — alternate-day steroids are preferred to minimize the negative effects on growth.
- Intra-articular steroid injections give benefit for 6–24 months
- DMARDs, e.g. methotrexate and sulfasalazine
- Combination therapy or biologics (e.g. anti-TNFα) may be required in refractory cases
- Surgery:
  — soft tissue release, osteotomies and joint replacement may be helpful.

Complications
- Loss of function and disability, e.g. secondary to stiff joints
- Chronic (bilateral) anterior uveitis is most severe in early-onset oligoarthritis with a positive ANA and/or HLA-DR5 titre:
  — can present with photophobia
  — may lead to blindness if regular check-ups and treatments are not carried out.
- Growth retardation often exacerbated by systemic steroid treatment
- Secondary amyloidosis
- Life disruption and depression.

CHAPTER 7

INJURY CLASSIFICATION AND PERIOPERATIVE CARE

INJURY ASSESSMENT, CLASSIFICATION AND TREATMENT

OVERVIEW OF INJURY ASSESSMENT

See Figure 7.1.

INITIAL ASSESSMENT

History

During the initial assessment of a suspected fracture or soft tissue injury it is important to determine the history of the injury (see Chapter 2), including the likely cause:

- Trauma causes damage of normal bone and soft tissue due to a direct or, more commonly, indirect force. It is useful to classify this in terms of the causative force, e.g. low velocity, high velocity or multiple (major) trauma
- Pathological, where the injury or fracture occurs in an already compromised, abnormally weak structure, e.g. a pathological fracture due to bone cysts, osteoporosis or bony metastasis
- Stress or fatigue, where repeated stress on the bone or surrounding soft tissue leads to injury, e.g. 2nd metatarsal neck fractures in army recruits ('march fracture') or golfer's elbow, respectively.

In all injuries, but particularly hand injuries, it is useful to determine the occupation and handedness of the patient. It is useful to ascertain from the patient what function they have lost as a result of their injury, as well as how this might have changed/worsened since the time of injury.

Examination (see Chapter 2)

Examine the affected and surrounding joint(s) and soft tissue for:

- Pain, bruising and tenderness
- Swelling, redness, heat or crepitus
- Range of movement (active and passive)
- Gross deformity, e.g. rotation, shortening or possible dislocation (a comparison with the unaffected limb can be helpful)
- Wounds for foreign bodies and potential soft tissue damage, e.g. nerves or tendons in open hand injuries
- Loss of function or sensation.

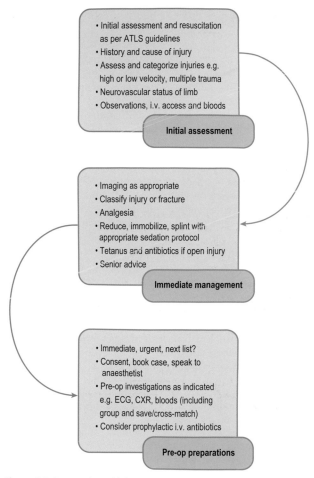

Figure 7.1 An overview of injury assessment. Local anaesthetic may be required to complete a thorough assessment, e.g. a ring block for a finger. Sensory deficit needs to be determined prior to this.

Neurovascular status

Assessment of the neurovascular status of the limb(s) is critical, and neglect at this stage can lead to avoidable complications. This includes examination of pulses, capillary refill time, colour and sensation distal to the injury site. Doppler may be used as part of the vascular assessment.

Some key examples of susceptible soft tissue injuries are as follows.

Nerves (see Chapter 4)
- Axillary: following a shoulder (anterior) dislocation and subsequent reduction, ± a proximal humeral fracture
- Radial: following a mid/distal shaft humeral or supracondylar fracture, elbow dislocation
- Posterior interosseous: following a Monteggia fracture-dislocation or isolated radial head or neck injury
- Ulnar: following supracondylar fractures of the humerus, elbow fracture-dislocation in adults or a wrist laceration
- Median: following supracondylar fractures of the humerus or a wrist laceration or fracture-dislocation
- Digital: following a medial or lateral laceration to the fingers or thumb (sensation and sweating are key features for testing)
- Sciatic: following a posterior hip dislocation or acetabular fracture
- Femoral: following a pubic ramus fracture
- Tibial: following a knee dislocation
- Common peroneal: following a fibular neck fracture or knee dislocation.

Blood vessels (division, compression, stretching, spasm)
- Axillary artery: following a shoulder dislocation
- Brachial artery: in supracondylar fractures of the humerus or following an elbow dislocation
- Radial artery: following a wrist laceration
- Ulnar artery: following a wrist laceration
- Digital artery: following a medial or lateral laceration to the fingers or thumb (if the artery is damaged it is probable that the nerve is damaged also)
- Femoral artery: following a fracture of the femur
- Lumbar–sacral plexus, iliac vessels or superior gluteal artery: following a pelvic fracture
- Popliteal artery: following a knee dislocation or proximal tibial fracture.

Muscles and tendons (sprain, rupture, division, crush, ischaemia with a limit of 6 hours for muscle)
- Long flexors and extensors to fingers (e.g. flexor digitorum superficialis, flexor digitorum profundus): following a wrist, hand or finger laceration
- Thumb flexors: following a wrist or thumb laceration
- Tendon sheath: direct contamination in palm or digital penetrating injury leading to infection (Figure 7.2)

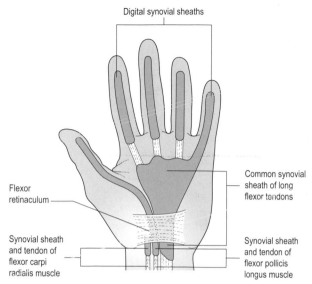

Figure 7.2 Penetrating injuries to the synovial sheaths of the hand can lead to infection spreading throughout the hand and proximally up the arm. Verdan's zones are used in assessing flexor tendon injury.

- EPL tendon: delayed rupture may occur after a Colles' fracture.

Imaging

Consider the appropriate imaging required at this point:

- Dependent on suspected injury and area(s) of body affected
- Radiographs may also be helpful to determine foreign body invasion of soft tissue
- Refer to local guidelines for appropriate indications
- Special reference should be made about the Ottawa Knee and Ankle Rules (see Chapter 3), which provide indications for imaging the knee and ankle, respectively.

CLASSIFICATION OF INJURY

Classification of fractures

The classification of paediatric injuries is discussed in Chapter 6.

Gustilo Classification		
I	Low energy, wound less than 1 cm	
II	Wound greater than 1 cm with moderate soft tissue damage	
III	High energy, wound greater than 1 cm with extensive soft tissue damage	
	IIIA	Adequate soft tissue cover
	IIIB	Inadequate soft tissue cover
	IIIC	Associated with arterial injury

Figure 7.3 Gustilo's classification of open fractures. An open wound fracture associated with farmyard injuries/highly contaminated wounds is classified grade III irrespective of the size of wound of soft tissue cover.

Classification of fractures by relation to surrounding tissue

- Simple or closed: fractures where the overlying skin is intact and the fracture site is not communicating with the skin or a body cavity
- Compound or open: fractures where there is significant soft tissue damage leading to broken ends communicating with the skin or body cavity. These are prone to infection and subsequent complications. They are classified according to Gustilo's classification of open fractures (Figure 7.3)
- Intra-articular: the fracture involves the joint/articulating surface, e.g. Bennett's fracture of the thumb.

Classification of fractures by shape (Figure 7.4)

- Transverse: caused by a direct blow, with the shape of the fractured bones allowing for better fracture alignment and union
- Spiral or oblique: are due to an indirect blow, e.g. twisting, and are unstable and difficult to align
- Sharp ends of a transverse, spiral or oblique fracture often cause damage to surrounding vessels and/or may break off ('butterfly fragment')
- Comminuted/multifragmented/complex: commonly due to severe direct trauma to the bone, a fracture of ≥2 parts, which is usually unstable
- Compression/crush: a fracture secondary to compression force, often in pathological bone, e.g. an osteoporotic vertebral crush fracture
- Avulsion: a fracture fragment, often secondary to a ligament being avulsed off bone, e.g. talus avulsion fracture secondary to an ankle dislocation.

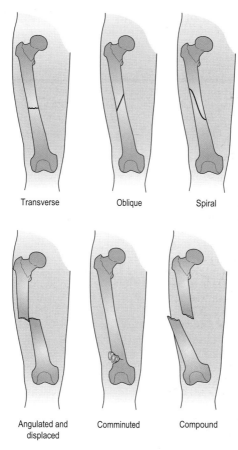

Figure 7.4 Fracture classification by shape and deformity.

Classification of fractures by deformity on radiograph (Figure 7.4)
- Displacement
- Rotation
- Angulation
- Shortening.

Classification of dislocations

By convention the direction of a dislocation, or fracture-dislocation, is determined by the position of the distal part relative to the proximal.

- Subluxation: when there is some, but incomplete loss of contact between articular surfaces of the joint. This type of injury may need active management to restore normal function
- Dislocation: when there is absolutely no contact between articular surfaces of the joint, e.g. anterior dislocation of the shoulder. Active treatment is needed
- Fracture-dislocation: when there is absolutely no contact between articular surfaces of the joint, with an associated periarticular fracture. Early management is more difficult in this situation, with removal of bony fragments from the joint space often needed. Fracture fixation and repair of surrounding ligaments may be required.

IMMEDIATE MANAGEMENT

See individual injury for the specific recommended management.

- Initial assessment and resuscitation should follow ATLS guidelines:
  — primary survey: **A**irway with C-spine control, **B**reathing and ventilation, **C**irculation with shock control, **D**isability, **E**xposure and environment. Within this, life-threatening injuries should be dealt with immediately. Monitor vitals at all times (pulse, BP, oxygen saturations, respiratory rate, GCS). Potential adjunctive imaging of the primary survey includes chest, C-spine and pelvic radiographs
  — secondary survey (when primary survey complete): including full body examination, appropriate further imaging (e.g. CT). The character and degree of the patient's injuries should now have been assessed.
- Analgesia (see Chapter 8)
- Wound management: an actively bleeding wound should be treated initially with direct pressure on the site
- Fractures and dislocations:
  — fluid resuscitation as blood loss, even in closed fractures, may be massive (Table 7.1)
  — immediate realignment of fractures using in-line traction, with immobilization in the anatomical position, will relieve

TABLE 7.1 Blood loss from different fracture sites	
Fracture site	*Blood loss (litres)*
Pelvis, hip	1.5–3
Femur to knee, humerus to elbow	1–2.5
Tibia to ankle, elbow to wrist	0.5–1.5

Adapted from Dandy & Edwards (2003).

    pain and reduce the risk of (further) soft tissue injury and/
    or bleeding
— open fractures will require a photograph, followed by
    covering with an iodine-soaked gauze and sterile dressing
— closed reduction is used to realign the bones to their
    anatomical position (this is done with appropriate
    analgesia and sedation); open reduction in theatre may be
    necessary. Remember to reassess neurovascular status pre
    and post reduction
— immobilization and/or traction for maintenance of position
    are achieved by back slab, plaster (e.g. plaster of Paris) or
    traction (e.g. Thomas splint); operative treatment may
    include internal (wires, plates, screws, intramedullary nails)
    or external fixation (e.g. Ilizarov frame) of the fracture.
● Tetanus and antibiotic prophylaxis should be given for open
   injuries (refer to local guidelines).

PREOPERATIVE MANAGEMENT

ASSESSMENT

Whether elective or emergency surgery is to be carried out, it is
important to undertake a thorough assessment before the
operation:

● History and examination (see Chapter 2)
● Co-morbidities:
   — establish the current health of the patient
   — determine the current control of any other medical
      problems, e.g. is their angina worse recently, is their
      insulin-dependant diabetes well controlled?
● Current medications (see below)
● Vital observations:
   — pulse, BP, oxygen saturations, respiratory rate.

- Investigations (refer to NICE guidelines and/or local guidelines for indications):
  — urinalysis
  — bloods, including group and save/cross-match
  — ECG
  — CXR.
- Full assessment of the affected limb for level of function, neurovascular status, infection and current analgesic requirements.

MEDICATIONS

Some drugs may need to be discontinued or altered before the operation. Senior advice in this matter, from the surgeon, anaesthetist or specialist physicians, will often need to be sought. Some examples to consider are as follows.

- Aspirin and clopidogrel:
  — these medications may need to be stopped 1–2 weeks before surgery, the decision often being anaesthetist (most importantly for spinal etc.), surgeon and patient dependent.
- Warfarin:
  — patients with heart valve replacements, recurrent DVTs or PEs may require conversion to i.v. heparin before the operation
  — patients on warfarin for atrial fibrillation may suffice with low molecular weight heparin (LMWH), e.g. enoxaparin.
- Nephrotoxic drugs, e.g. ACE inhibitors, NSAIDs:
  — patients susceptible to developing acute renal failure postoperatively may need some medications temporarily stopped. Such patients may benefit from early catheterization to monitor urine output.
- Antihypertensives:
  — patients will often have to remain on these medications for the operation.
- Steroids:
  — patients on long-term oral steroids may require supplementation with increased doses of hydrocortisone perioperatively.
- Consider an insulin sliding scale for insulin-dependent diabetic patients (mandatory when fasting).

It is important to consider prophylaxis for avoidable complications preoperatively (patient, operation and injury dependent):

open wounds always

- Antibiotics:
  — refer to local guidelines for current indications.
- DVT/PE:
  — TED stockings as mechanical prophylaxis if there are palpable pedal pulses or reasonable ankle–brachial pressure indices (ABPIs)
  — subcutaneous LMWH
  — antiplatelet agent, e.g. aspirin, with or without LMWH.

POSTOPERATIVE MANAGEMENT AND COMPLICATIONS

POSTOPERATIVE ASSESSMENT AND MEDICAL COMPLICATIONS

Regular monitoring of vital observations (pulse, BP, urine output, respiratory rate, oxygen saturations and temperature) and bloods is an essential part of the immediate postoperative period. The Scottish Early Warning Scoring (SEWS) chart is an example of an effective way of identifying ill patients. System management includes the following:

- Cardiovascular and renal assessment:
  — patients should be warm and well perfused
  — monitor for causes and signs of shock, e.g. hypovolaemia due to bleeding from the operative site or from the GI tract (secondary to NSAIDs), sepsis, cardiogenic shock
  — monitor fluid and electrolyte balance regularly (urine output >0.5 ml/kg/h)
  — patients with pre-existing renal disease should be on a strict fluid balance
  — susceptible patients are those with pre-existing IHD, cardiovascular risk factors, the elderly and those with chronic kidney disease
  — potential complications include atrial fibrillation, myocardial infarction, pulmonary oedema, acute renal failure, urinary tract infection, urinary retention.
- Respiratory assessment:
  — monitor for symptoms and signs of respiratory distress, e.g. pyrexia, productive cough, abnormal CXR, increasing respiratory rate and/or oxygen requirements
  — susceptible patients are those with pre-existing pulmonary disease, e.g. chronic obstructive pulmonary disease (COPD)

— potential complications include pulmonary oedema,
pulmonary embolus, pneumonia, ARDS, atelectasis.
- Systemic assessment:
— monitor for sepsis, systemic inflammatory response
syndrome (SIRS) and disseminated intravascular
coagulation (DIC)
— nutritional intake should be monitored as soon as possible
postoperatively, with advice sought early if calorie
requirements are not being met
— in relation to nutrition, postoperative ileus may complicate
oral intake due to abdominal pain and distension, along
with vomiting.
- Operative field assessment:
— neurovascular assessment of the limb(s) operated on
— postoperative radiographs
— early physiotherapy and occupational therapy input.
- Analgesia assessment:
— analgesic ladder (see Chapter 8)
— some patients will require strong analgesia, e.g. morphine
patient-controlled analgesia (PCA) or epidurals.

Immediate assessment of the complications listed above will
include:

- Bloods, e.g. for anaemia, renal failure, infection, hepatic shock
- ABGs, e.g. to determine hypoxia or degree of acidaemia/
alkalaemia
- ECG, e.g. for signs of myocardial ischaemia or dysrhythmia
- CXR, e.g. for signs of consolidation or fluid overload
- Septic screen, e.g. sputum culture to determine organism
causing pneumonia.

Early specialist guidance and higher levels of care, e.g.
HDU/ITU, may be required to deal with these potentially
life-threatening complications.

FRACTURE COMPLICATIONS

The fracture healing process takes approximately 8–10 weeks (less
in children):

1. Fracture haematoma
2. Inflammation (vascular invasion, inflammatory mediators,
granulation tissue)
3. Repair (subperiosteal osteoblast stimulation, endochondral and
intramembranous ossification, bone matrix formation)

TABLE 7.2 Complications of fractures and when they commonly occur post injury

	Complications
Instant	Neurovascular compromise Soft tissue injury Organ injury due to hypovolaemia (bleeding)
Early	Infection, e.g. at wound site, LRTI, ARDS Renal dysfunction, e.g. retention or failure Emboli, e.g. DVT, PE, fat embolus DIC Fracture related, e.g. nerve damage due to poor cast position, failure of reduction, compartment syndrome
Delayed	Osteoarthritis Avascular necrosis Sudeck's atrophy Myositis ossificans Disunion, deformity, stiffness and contracture

LRTI, lower respiratory tract infection.

4. Remodelling (fusiform callus → woven bone → lamellar bone).

If the fracture is untreated or managed incorrectly, one of the following is likely to occur as a delayed complication.

- Delayed union: a fracture that takes longer than expected to unite and heal due to organic (e.g. poor vascular supply due to compartment syndrome, soft tissue injury and infection) or mechanical (poor splint) insufficiency
- Non-union: non-united bone is the product if the healing process has been unsuccessful; this may be atrophic with thinning bone ends indicative of an avascular blood supply and no more bone growth, or hypertrophic with expanded bone ends indicative of instability but continuing bone growth
- Malunion: here the fracture has healed and the bone is united, but not in the correct position due to displacement (shortening, translation, rotation or angulation) and/or poor fracture position management; sometimes the subsequent deformity is of no functional consequence or can lead to OA.

There are numerous other significant complications (Table 7.2) which may occur with or without an operative intervention. Five complications of particular importance are shown below.

Fat embolism

- An uncommon complication that usually occurs in the first week after a long bone injury, e.g. femoral shaft fracture
- Two possible causes are:
  - direct embolization of lipid globules from bone marrow adipocytes of the medullary canal at the fracture site
  - altered response of lipid metabolism secondary to injury, which generates numerous small fat particles.
- The result is embolization of small fat globules to the end blood vessels in organs throughout the body (often the lung)
- Signs depend on the end-organ affected and include:
  - shortness of breath, hypoxia, tachycardia, neurological upset (confusion, seizures, coma), ARDS if severe, ARF, petechial haemorrhagic rash and pyrexia.
- Investigations include:
  - bloods (thrombocytopenia)
  - urine and sputum analysis (lipids may be seen)
  - ABG (low pO_2)
  - CXR (peripheral patchy consolidation).
- Treatment is with oxygen, steroids, i.v. fluids and organ support
- Prevention is with early stabilization and immobilization of the fracture.

Compartment syndrome

- Common after:
  - lower leg and forearm fractures (open or closed)
  - tight casts
  - burns and crush injuries.
- Injured tissue expands due to oedema, haemorrhage and/or infection. As there is limited space within the enclosed fascial compartment, intracompartmental pressure rises, vascular (arterial and venous) flow is impaired, and the tissue (muscle and nerve) becomes ischaemic and necrotic. With muscle this causes fibrosis and permanent contracture of the muscle (Volkmann's ischaemic contracture)
- Commonly presents with intense and severe pain, which is refractory to analgesia, out of proportion and worse on passive stretch. Paralysis, paraesthesia, pallor and absent pulses are very late signs

- Compartment monitors can be used to monitor pressures (diagnostic if diastolic blood pressure − intracompartmental pressure is ≤30 mmHg).
- Treatment is with:
  — maintenance of BP
  — cast removal (if appropriate)
  — early open surgical decompression fasciotomy.

Crush syndrome

- Crushing, ischaemia and/or necrosis of muscle (often large muscle, e.g. thigh):
  — leads to release of myoglobin into the circulation due to muscle breakdown (rhabdomyolysis).
- Common findings include:
  — myoglobinuria, which leads to dark urine
  — raised CK level and deranged U&Es
  — metabolic acidosis
  — hypovolaemia, acute renal failure
  — disseminated intravascular coagulation (DIC)
  — beware of compartment syndrome.
- Treatment is with:
  — intensive organ support, aggressive i.v. fluids with strict fluid balance
  — diuretics and urine alkalization
  — dialysis if severe enough
  — amputation may be needed.

Avascular necrosis

- When a fracture affects the vascular supply to a bone and/or joint, bone ischaemia, necrosis and death occur
- It is found commonly when the vascular supply of the bone originates from the medullary cavity. Common susceptible injuries are:
  — a proximal pole scaphoid fracture as the vascular supply to the bone enters through the distal edge
  — an intracapsular femoral neck fracture when the retinacular vessels that supply the head of the femur are interrupted
  — a neck of talus fracture as the vascular supply enters the bone via the talus neck
  — a lunate dislocation.

- Patients present with a destroyed, stiff and painful joint, which can take years to develop
- Diagnosis is confirmed when an avascular fragment appears more dense than surrounding bone on a radiograph due to collapse, calcification and osteoporosis. Chondrolysis is seen on MRI
- Treatment is with a combination of:
  — analgesia and bed rest
  — surgery (joint replacement or fusion).
- Prevention is with:
  — early reduction and definitive treatment.

THERAPEUTICS

We recommend that the first point of reference when prescribing is the BNF. Some of these medications will be used in community practice and in other specialities. The aim of this chapter is to provide detailed information on the drugs commonly used within orthopaedics and rheumatology.

The drug tables in this chapter were originally published in *Churchill's In Clinical Practice Series: Rheumatology*, Churchill Livingstone, 2004, Panayi and Dickson, ISBN 9780443074677. Updated by kind permission of Dr John Dickson.

ANALGESIA (Tables 8.1–8.3)

- Pain control is an essential part of any surgical or medical speciality
- WHO's Pain Relief Ladder (Figure 8.1) is a useful tool when trying to decide what analgesia is appropriate to prescribe, whether it is within the acute (e.g. postoperative) or chronic (e.g. arthritis) setting
- COX-2 is primarily present at sites of inflammation, producing prostaglandins, which leads to the sensation of pain (Figure 8.2)
- Selective inhibitors of COX-2 are equally as effective in controlling pain and inflammation as the non-selective NSAIDs that inhibit both COX-1 and COX-2, and are less

TABLE 8.1 Paracetamol	
Uses	Mild to moderate pain Pyrexia
Mechanism of action	Uncertain; possibly reduces the CNS formation of prostaglandins via inhibition of a COX variant Effective analgesic, but less effective than NSAIDs as an anti-inflammatory Favoured in the elderly as it does not precipitate GI upset, cardiac failure or renal impairment
Side effects	Rash (rare), haematological disorders (rare) Hepatic failure in overdose
Contraindication/caution	No absolute contraindications Caution in hepatic or renal impairment
Recommended dose	0.5–1 g 4–6 hourly, max. 4 g/24 h
Routes of administration	Oral, rectal, i.v.

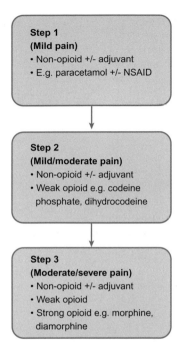

Figure 8.1 Analgesia should be prescribed using the above step-wise regimen. Adjuvant therapies include splints, acupuncture, physiotherapy etc. (Adapted from the WHO's Pain Relief Ladder.)

likely to cause GI upset. However, the risk of cardiovascular disease seems to be increased with all NSAIDs and these drugs are contraindicated in patients with pre-existing cardiovascular disease
- Topical NSAIDs can be helpful in some patients with soft tissue rheumatism and osteoarthritis and are less likely to cause systemic side effects
- Risk factors for developing gastric or, less commonly, duodenal ulcers due to NSAID use are:
  — a history of ulcers or GI bleeds (potential for perforation or bleeding from an established ulcer)
  — being elderly, as this group often has significant co-morbidities
  — associated steroid or anticoagulant use, e.g. prednisolone or aspirin

TABLE 8.2 NSAIDs (COX inhibitors), e.g. ibuprofen, diclofenac, celecoxib

Uses	Inflammatory arthritis (RA, AS, PsA) Osteoarthritis Bone metastases Perioperative pain Pyrexia
Mechanism of action	Reversible inhibition of COX, which decreases the production of prostaglandins (Figure 8.2) and reduces inflammation Non-selective NSAIDs also inhibit COX-1, which is important for protection of the GI mucosa
Side effects	GI upset and peptic ulceration (less likely with COX-2 selective drugs) Renal impairment, fluid retention and hypertension Increased risk of cardiovascular disease Hypersensitivity, e.g. rash, bronchospasm May have an inhibitory effect on bone healing
Contraindication/caution	ARF, CRF, IHD, CCF, asthma (~10%), coagulopathies Pregnancy, breast feeding, elderly
Recommended dose	Ibuprofen: 400 mg 8 hourly, max. 1.2 g/24 h Diclofenac: 50 mg 8 hourly, max. 150 mg/24 h Celecoxib: 100 mg bd, max. 400 mg/24 h
Routes of administration	Ibuprofen: oral, topical Diclofenac: oral, rectal, i.m., i.v., topical Celecoxib: oral

CCF, congestive cardiac failure; CRF, chronic renal failure.

— high-risk NSAID use, e.g. large doses or more than one type prescribed.
- In the presence of these risk factors, gastric protection should be considered with a PPI, e.g. omeprazole 20 mg once daily:
  — lack of symptoms does *not* mean there is no ulcer
  — if ulceration or bleeding is thought likely, stopping all potentially causative medications, prescribing a high-dose PPI and organizing an upper GI endoscopy should all be considered (refer to local guidelines)

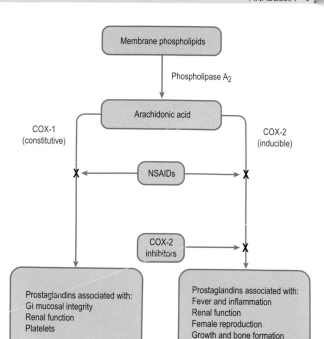

NSAID = nonsteroidal anti-inflammatory drug;
COX = cyclo-oxygenase;
GI = gastrointestinal

Figure 8.2 Cyclo-oxygenase (COX) is an enzyme that converts arachidonic acid into prostaglandins. NSAIDs inhibit this action.

— a significant GI bleed will require establishment of haemodynamic stability, often with fluid resuscitation, followed by an urgent upper GI endoscopy.
● Nausea and vomiting, as well as constipation, are common side effects of opiate use. Therefore, it is useful to prescribe antiemetics and laxatives as required:
— for constipation: senna 7.5–15 mg at night
— for nausea and vomiting: metoclopramide 10 mg 8 hourly.
● Opiate toxicity is characterized by hallucinations (e.g. spiders), respiratory depression, a reduced conscious level (low GCS)

TABLE 8.3 Opiates (opioid receptor agonists)

Uses	Mild to severe pain (aim for short-term use where possible)
Mechanism of action	Decrease pain via binding to opioid receptors (mu, delta, kappa in order of affinity) within central and peripheral nervous system, as well as spinal cord
Side effects	Nausea and vomiting Constipation Drowsiness and respiratory depression Hypotension Confusion, particularly in the elderly
Contraindication/caution	Patients with a low or fluctuating GCS, e.g. stroke, head injury Acute respiratory depression or failure Acute alcohol excess, paralytic ileus, hepatic or renal impairment Pregnancy, breast feeding, elderly
Recommended dose	Codeine phosphate: 30–60 mg 4 hourly, max. 240 mg/24 h Dihydrocodeine tartrate: 30 mg 4–6 hourly Tramadol HCl: 50–100 mg 4–6 hourly, max. 400 mg/24 h Morphine salts: dependent on route and indication (see BNF)
Routes of administration	Codeine phosphate: oral, i.m. Dihydrocodeine tartrate: oral, i.m., s.c. Tramadol HCl: oral, i.m., i.v. Morphine salts: oral, rectal, i.m., s.c., i.v.

and pinpoint pupils. The short-acting opioid antagonist naloxone can be used to reverse toxicity

- Dependence and tolerance are potential adverse effects of opiates when used recreationally or in the chronic setting, respectively. Withdrawal signs are GI upset, sweating, insomnia, tremor and yawning
- Compound analgesics, e.g. co-codamol and co-dydramol, are combinations of a first-step analgesic, e.g. paracetamol, with a weak opioid, e.g. codeine. They often come in various dose combinations:
  — co-codamol 8/500 = 500 mg paracetamol + 8 mg codeine phosphate; normal dosing is 2 tablets every 6 hours with a maximum of 8 tablets per day
  — the same side effects and contraindications/cautions as those described under paracetamol and opiates apply.

STEROIDS (Table 8.4)

- The anti-inflammatory and immunosuppressive properties of corticosteroids make them valuable agents for the treatment of systemic inflammatory disease. Local steroid injections are also used widely in the treatment of soft tissue rheumatism (e.g. tennis elbow, golfer's elbow), OA and in patients with inflammatory arthritis where a single joint is predominantly affected
- When systemic steroids are required, the maintenance dose should be as low as is necessary to maintain symptom control or control of inflammation
- Steroid-sparing agents (e.g. azathioprine) are often used in addition to steroids when the maintenance prednisolone dose cannot be reduced below 10–15 mg/24 h
- Higher doses (40–80 mg prednisolone daily) may be required during induction of remission or relapse in patients with vasculitis, SLE and other inflammatory diseases

TABLE 8.4 Steroids

Uses	Rheumatoid arthritis SLE, vasculitis, polymyositis and dermatomyositis Giant cell arthritis/PMR
Mechanism of action	Multiple, including inhibition of macrophages and T and B lymphocytes
Side effects	Hypertension, weight gain, fluid retention, skin changes (e.g. thin), osteoporosis, alteration of mood, peptic ulcers, acute pancreatitis, Cushing's syndrome, diabetes, myopathy, growth disturbance (children)
Contraindication/caution	Systemic infection Renal, liver or heart failure Peptic ulcers, acute pancreatitis Cushing's syndrome, diabetes, hypertension, osteoporosis Pregnancy, breast feeding, elderly, children
Recommended dose	Dependent on route and indication (see BNF).
Routes of administration	Prednisolone: oral, i.m. Hydrocortisone: oral, i.m., i.v. Hydrocortisone acetate: intra-articular, soft tissue

- Patients on long-term steroids require an increase in their maintenance dose at the time of concomitant illness or stress (e.g. surgery)
- Long-term steroid use can lead to osteoporosis, and prophylaxis should be contemplated in these patients (see 'Prevention and treatment of osteoporosis', below).

DISEASE-MODIFYING ANTIRHEUMATIC DRUGS (DMARDS) (Tables 8.5–8.15)

- DMARDs are gradual-onset anti-inflammatory agents that improve and control symptoms whilst also slowing disease progression (to varying degrees)
- They are often prescribed by a specialist, i.e. a consultant rheumatologist
- Combinations may be used for the treatment of RA
- Bone marrow suppression, e.g. neutropenia leading to infection, or thrombocytopenia leading to bruising, is a common side effect of many of these drugs. It is essential to monitor all DMARDs for evidence of toxicity, with dose

TABLE 8.5 Azathioprine	
Uses	Rheumatoid arthritis Seronegative spondyloarthritis, e.g. PsA SLE and vasculitis Giant cell arthritis/PMR
Mechanism of action	A cytotoxic agent that inhibits DNA synthesis, thereby causing immunosuppression
Side effects	Bone marrow suppression Alopecia GI upset, e.g. nausea, vomiting, diarrhoea Deranged LFTs, e.g. hepatitis, cholestatic jaundice Herpes zoster
Contraindication/caution	Hypersensitivity Breast feeding Hepatic or renal impairment Pregnancy, elderly
Recommended dose	1–3 mg/kg/24 h
Routes of administration	Oral, i.v.

TABLE 8.6 Cyclophosphamide

Uses	SLE Vasculitis RA with systemic manifestations
Mechanism of action	An alkylating agent that forms cross-links between strands of DNA, halting cell replication and division, thereby causing immunosuppression
Side effects	GI upset, e.g. nausea, vomiting, weight loss Bone marrow suppression Alopecia Haemorrhagic cystitis*, azoospermia, anovulation
Contraindication/caution	Porphyria Hepatic or renal impairment Pregnancy (teratogenic), breast feeding
Recommended dose	Oral: 1–2 mg/kg/24 h Intravenous: 0.5–1 g/month
Routes of administration	Oral, i.v.

* Patients receiving high-dose i.v. cyclophosphamide should be prescribed mesna and be advised to take large volumes of fluid to reduce the risk of this complication.

reduction as appropriate. This is done using one, or more, of the following:
— bloods: FBC, U&Es, LFTs
— urinalysis: protein and blood
— BP
— eye examination including fundoscopy.

TABLE 8.7 Ciclosporin

Uses	Rheumatoid arthritis Seronegative spondyloarthritis, e.g. PsA
Mechanism of action	An immunosuppressive agent that reduces inflammation by inhibiting T cells and decreasing the production of IL-2
Side effects	GI upset Malignant or refractory hypertension Renal or hepatic dysfunction with the potential for toxicity, leading to electrolyte, lipid and sugar disturbances Gout, gum hypertrophy
Contraindication/caution	Porphyria Malignant or refractory hypertension Hepatic or renal impairment, e.g. nephrotic syndrome Pregnancy, breast feeding
Recommended dose	2.5–4 mg/kg/24 h
Route of administration	Oral

IL, interleukin.

TABLE 8.8 Gold

Uses	Rheumatoid arthritis
Mechanism of action	Unknown, but has effects on polymorphs, macrophages and lymphocytes and inhibits synovial cell proliferation
Side effects	Bone marrow suppression Alopecia GI upset, e.g. diarrhoea, colitis Renal dysfunction (glomerulonephritis) Deranged LFTs, e.g. cholestatic jaundice, toxicity Dermatitis, pruritic rash, oral ulcers, pulmonary fibrosis
Contraindication/caution	SLE, porphyria, pulmonary fibrosis IBD, necrotizing enterocolitis Hypersensitivity with pre-existing skin disorders Hepatic or renal impairment Pregnancy, breast feeding, elderly
Recommended dose	Auranofin: 6 mg/24 h Sodium aurothiomalate: 10 mg test dose, then 50 mg/week
Routes of administration	Auranofin: oral Sodium aurothiomalate: i.m.

TABLE 8.9 Hydroxychloroquine

Uses	Rheumatoid arthritis SLE
Mechanism of action	Inhibits lysozyme function and antigen processing
Side effects	Eye toxicity (retinopathy) with long-term use GI upset, e.g. nausea, vomiting, diarrhoea, weight loss Pruritic rash, headache, skin and hair changes/discoloration Bone marrow suppression
Contraindication/caution	Alcohol excess Hepatic or renal impairment Epilepsy, myasthenia gravis, psoriasis, porphyria Pregnancy, breast feeding, elderly
Recommended dose	200–400 mg/24 h
Route of administration	Oral

TABLE 8.10 Leflunomide

Uses	Rheumatoid arthritis Psoriatic arthritis
Mechanism of action	An agent that specifically inhibits DNA synthesis in lymphocytes, thereby causing immunosuppression
Side effects	GI upset, e.g. nausea, vomiting, diarrhoea, weight loss Hypertension, headaches, tenosynovitis Alopecia, rash Bone marrow suppression Renal or hepatic dysfunction
Contraindication/caution	Bone marrow dysfunction, immunosuppressed patient Hepatic (potential for toxicity) or renal impairment Pregnancy* (teratogenic), breast feeding
Recommended dose	Loading: 100 mg/24 h for 3 days Maintenance: 10–20 mg/24 h
Route of administration	Oral

* Contraception is essential during and after treatment for both men and women.

TABLE 8.11 Methotrexate

Uses	Rheumatoid arthritis Vasculitides Connective tissue disease, e.g. SLE Seronegative spondyloarthritis, e.g. PsA
Mechanism of action	A cytotoxic agent that inhibits DNA synthesis by inhibiting dihydrofolate reductase, thereby causing immunosuppression
Side effects	GI upset, e.g. ulcers, bleeding, weight loss, diarrhoea, toxic colon Hepatic toxicity and potentially cirrhosis, renal failure Acute pneumonitis, pulmonary fibrosis or oedema Hypersensitivity, GU disturbances Rash, joint and muscle pain, precipitation of vasculitis Bone marrow suppression, alopecia
Contraindication/caution	Bone marrow dysfunction, immunosuppressed patient GI dysfunction, e.g. PUD, IBD Hepatic or renal impairment, alcohol excess Pregnancy* (teratogenic), breast feeding Patients with ascites or pleural effusions
Recommended dose	7.5 mg/week Often given with 5 mg of folic acid to reduce side effects
Routes of administration	Oral, s.c., i.m., i.v., intrathecal

GU, genitourinary; PUD, peptic ulcer disease.
* Contraception is essential during and after treatment for both men and women.

TABLE 8.12 Penicillamine

Uses	Rheumatoid arthritis
Mechanism of action	Unknown, but various actions on monocytes, lymphocytes and T cells demonstrated in vitro
Side effects	GI upset, e.g. nausea, vomiting, weight loss Reversible taste loss, mouth ulcers Proteinuria (nephrotic syndrome, nephritis) Lupus erythematosus-type and myasthenia gravis-type syndromes Bone marrow suppression, fever Alopecia, rash, gynaecomastia
Contraindication/caution	SLE Hepatic or renal impairment Current nephrotoxic medications or gold therapy Pregnancy Allergy to penicillin
Recommended dose	250–750 mg/24 h (before food)
Route of administration	Oral

TABLE 8.13 Sulfasalazine

Uses	Rheumatoid arthritis Seronegative spondarthritis
Mechanism of action	Incompletely understood, but scavenges proinflammatory reactive oxygen species and reduces T cell activation
Side effects	GI upset, e.g. nausea, abdominal pain, weight loss Acute pancreatitis, renal or hepatic dysfunction Rash, lupus erythematosus-type syndrome Bone marrow suppression Urine discoloration (orange), infertility (reversible)
Contraindication/caution	Renal or hepatic impairment Hypersensitivity Porphyria Toddlers
Recommended dose	500 mg/24 h after food (enteric-coated), increasing gradually to 3–4 g/24 h in divided doses
Routes of administration	Oral, rectal

TABLE 8.14 Anti-TNF therapy (infliximab, etanercept, adalimumab)

Uses	Inflammatory arthritis (RA, AS, PsA)
Mechanism of action	Blocks effects of the proinflammatory cytokine TNFα, thereby reducing inflammation
Side effects	GI upset, e.g. nausea, vomiting, oesophagitis, bleeding Renal dysfunction Hypotension, myocardial or cerebral ischaemia, VTE Rash, fever, seizures, lymphadenopathy, infection Increased risk of malignancy
Contraindication/caution	Acute infection, herpes zoster, immunosuppressed patient Possibility of TB (active or latent) Pregnancy* (teratogenic), breast feeding Cardiac failure
Recommended dose	See BNF
Routes of administration	i.v., s.c.

* Contraception is essential during and after treatment for both men and women.

TABLE 8.15 Anti-B cell therapy (rituximab)

Uses	Rheumatoid arthritis SLE
Mechanism of action	Causes apoptosis of B cells, thereby causing immunosuppression
Side effects	Rash, fever Infusion reaction (pre-dose steroids may help)
Contraindication/caution	Cardiovascular disease Pregnancy, breast feeding
Recommended dose	See BNF
Route of administration	i.v.

PREVENTION AND TREATMENT OF OSTEOPOROSIS (Tables 8.16–8.21)

- Calcium and vitamin D preparations should be considered in all patients at risk of developing osteoporosis and where a deficiency is likely:
  — they are often used as adjunct to the medications shown below
  — GI upset and hypercalcaemia are the most common complications associated with these drugs.
- Lifestyle changes are essential, e.g. stopping smoking
- Calcitonin, via a nasal spray, is a potential alternative when bisphosphonates are not tolerated.

TABLE 8.16 Calcitonin	
Uses	Osteoporosis Paget's disease Bone metastases
Mechanism of action	Osteoclast inhibitor that prevents postmenopausal bone loss Reduces risk of vertebral fractures Potential analgesic effects
Side effects	GI upset, e.g. nausea, vomiting, diarrhoea, pain ENT upset (with nasal spray), e.g. rhinitis, epistaxis, sinusitis Headache, dizziness Hypersensitivity
Contraindication/caution	Hypersensitivity Renal impairment Cardiac failure Pregnancy, breast feeding
Recommended dose	Intranasal spray for osteoporosis: 200 U/24 h sc for osteoporosis: 100 U/24 h
Routes of administration	Intranasal spray, s.c.

ENT = ear, nose and throat.

TABLE 8.17 Parathyroid hormone (teriparatide)

Uses	Osteoporosis
Mechanism of action	A recombinant that stimulates bone formation Reduces risk of vertebral and non-vertebral fractures
Side effects	GI upset, e.g. nausea, GORD, haemorrhoids GU upset, e.g. polyuria Postural hypotension, dizziness, vertigo Depression, sciatica
Contraindication/caution	Pre-existing bone disorders, e.g. Paget's Hypercalcaemia, hyperparathyroidism, raised ALP History of radiation to bone Pregnancy, breast feeding
Recommended dose	20 µg/24 h (period of 18 months max.)
Route of administration	s.c.

GORD, gastro-oesophageal reflux disease; GU, genitourinary.

TABLE 8.18 Strontium ranelate

Uses	Osteoporosis
Mechanism of action	Reduces bone turnover (inhibits osteoclastic bone resorption) and prevents postmenopausal bone loss Reduces risk of vertebral and non-vertebral fractures
Side effects	GI upset, e.g. nausea, diarrhoea Skin upset, e.g. eczema, dermatitis Headache Increased risk of VTE
Contraindication/caution	History of VTE, coagulopathies Renal impairment
Recommended dose	2 g once at night in water (avoid food)
Route of administration	Oral

TABLE 8.19 Hormone replacement therapy

Uses	Osteoporosis
Mechanism of action	Prevents postmenopausal bone loss by inhibiting bone remodelling Reduces risk of vertebral and non-vertebral fractures
Side effects	Fluid retention, weight gain, menstrual disturbance Increased risk of breast and endometrial cancer, DVT, stroke, cardiovascular disease
Contraindication/caution	Breast cancer, endometrial cancer History of VTE, coagulopathies Hepatic impairment Pregnancy, breast feeding
Recommended dose	See BNF
Routes of administration	Oral, transdermal, depot

TABLE 8.20 Selective oestrogen receptor modulators (SERMs), e.g. raloxifene

Uses	Osteoporosis
Mechanism of action	Partial oestrogen receptor agonist that reduces bone turnover (inhibits osteoclastic bone resorption) and prevents postmenopausal bone loss Reduces the risk of vertebral fractures
Side effects	Hot flushes, insomnia, muscle cramps, fluid retention Increased risk of VTE GI upset Hypertension, headache, rash
Contraindication/caution	Breast cancer*, endometrial cancer History of VTE, coagulopathies Hepatic or renal impairment Pregnancy, breast feeding
Recommended dose	60 mg/24 h
Route of administration	Oral

* Although this is listed as a caution, data from clinical trials show that long-term use of raloxifene is associated with a significantly reduced risk of breast cancer.

TABLE 8.21 Bisphosphonates, e.g. alendronic acid (alendronate), risedronate, zoledronic acid (zoledronate)

Uses	Osteoporosis Paget's disease Bone metastases
Mechanism of action	Pyrophosphate analogues that are adsorbed into bone, decreasing bone turnover Reduce risk of vertebral and non-vertebral fractures in osteoporosis Help bone pain in Paget's disease Reduce the risk of skeletal complication in patients with metastatic bone disease
Side effects	GI upset, e.g. pain, dyspepsia, reflux, diarrhoea, melaena Oesophageal upset, e.g. ulcers, strictures, inflammation Headache, rash, skin changes, uveitis, scleritis Hypersensitivity Hypocalcaemia (with i.v. use) Osteonecrosis of the jaw (rare)
Contraindication/caution	Dysphagia, stricture, achalasia Pregnancy, breast feeding, hypocalcaemia GI ulceration, inflammation or bleeding Renal impairment
Recommended dose	Depends on drug and indication. See BNF
Route of administration	Oral

GOUT (Tables 8.22–8.23)

- Acute attacks can be controlled with a combination of NSAIDs, colchicine, systemic corticosteroids or intra-articular corticosteroids
- Colchicine or NSAID cover is often required as prophylaxis against flares during initiation of urate-lowering therapy (e.g. allopurinol). Allopurinol should not be commenced during an acute attack
- A sufficient fluid intake is essential
- Lifestyle changes are essential, e.g. reduce alcohol intake.

TABLE 8.22 Colchicine

Uses	Acute gout attack
Mechanism of action	Inhibits neutrophil migration and function
Side effects	GI upset, e.g. nausea, vomiting, diarrhoea (titrate dose to frequency), bleeding Bone marrow suppression Renal or hepatic dysfunction
Contraindication/caution	Pregnancy, breast feeding, elderly Renal, hepatic or cardiac impairment
Recommended dose	500 µg 4 hourly, max. 6 mg per course
Route of administration	Oral

TABLE 8.23 Allopurinol

Uses	Long-term prevention and control of gout
Mechanism of action	Inhibits xanthine oxidase, thereby decreasing the production of uric acid
Side effects	Rash, hypersensitivity GI upset Headache, hypertension Hepatic impairment with the potential for toxicity Bone marrow suppression
Contraindication/caution	Acute gout (can cause exacerbation) Pregnancy, breast feeding Renal or hepatic impairment
Recommended dose	100–300 mg/24 h (after food)
Route of administration	Oral

BIBLIOGRAPHY,
FURTHER READING
AND USEFUL
WEBSITES

BIBLIOGRAPHY AND FURTHER READING

Aids to the Examination of the Peripheral Nervous System, 4th ed. Edinburgh: Saunders; 2000.

American College of Surgeons Committee on Trauma. ATLS Student Course Manual, 7th ed. Chicago: American College of Surgeons; 2004.

Ballinger A, Patchett S. Saunders' Pocket Essentials of Clinical Medicine, 3rd ed. Edinburgh: Saunders; 2003.

Boon NA, Colledge NR, Walker BR, Hunter JAA. Davidson's Principles and Practice of Medicine, 20th ed. Edinburgh: Churchill Livingstone; 2006.

British National Formulary: Current Edition

Bucholz RW, Heckman JD. Rockwood and Green's Fractures in Adults, 6th ed. Philadelphia: Lippincott Williams and Wilkins; 2005.

Collier J, Longmore M, Scally P. Oxford Handbook of Clinical Specialities, 6th ed. Oxford: Oxford University Press; 2003.

Coote A, Haslam P. Crash Course: Rheumatology and Orthopaedics. Edinburgh: Mosby; 2004.

Cotran RS, Kumar V, Collins T. Robbins Pathologic Basis of Disease, 6th ed. Philadelphia: Saunders; 1999:1215–1269.

Dandy DJ, Edwards DJ. Essential Orthopaedics and Trauma, 4th ed. Elsevier: Churchill Livingstone; 2003.

Davey P. Medicine at a Glance. Oxford: Blackwell Science; 2002.

Drake R, Vogl W, Mitchell A. Gray's Anatomy for Students. Edinburgh: Churchill Livingstone; 2005.

Dykes M, Ameerally P. Crash Course: Anatomy, 2nd ed. Edinburgh: Mosby; 2002.

Ford MJ, Hennessay I, Japp A. Introduction to Clinical Examination, 8th ed. Edinburgh: Churchill Livingstone; 2005.

Fuller G, Manford M. Neurology: An Illustrated Colour Text. Edinburgh: Churchill Livingstone; 2000.

Gosling JA, Harris PF, Humpherson JR, Whitmore L, Willan PLT. Human Anatomy: Color Atlas and Text, 4th ed. Edinburgh: Mosby; 2002.

Gray's Anatomy, 38th ed. Edinburgh: Churchill Livingstone; 1995.

Gunn C. Bones and Joints: A Guide for Students, 4th ed. Edinburgh: Churchill Livingstone; 2002.

Haslett C, Chilvers ER, Boon NA, Colledge NR. Davidson's Principles and Practice of Medicine, 19th ed. Edinburgh: Churchill Livingstone; 2002.

Kumar P, Clark M. Clinical Medicine, 6th ed. Edinburgh: Saunders; 2005.

Maddison PJ, Isenberg DA, Woo P, Glass DN. Oxford Textbook of Rheumatology, 2nd ed. Oxford: Oxford University Press; 1998.

McLatchie GR, Leaper DJ. Oxford Handbook of Clinical Surgery, 2nd ed. Oxford: Oxford University Press; 2002.

McRae R. Clinical Orthopaedic Examination, 5th ed. Edinburgh: Churchill Livingstone; 2004.

McRae R. Pocketbook of Orthopaedics and Fractures, 2nd ed. Edinburgh: Churchill Livingstone; 2006.

Moore KL, Agur AMR. Essential Clinical Anatomy. Baltimore: Williams and Wilkins; 1995.

Munro JF, Campbell IW. MacLeod's Clinical Examination, 10th ed. Edinburgh: Churchill Livingstone; 2000.

Page CP, Curtis MJ, Sutter MC, Walker MJA. Integrated pharmacology. London: Mosby; 1997.

Parchment-Smith C. Essential revision notes for intercollegiate MRCS Book 2, 1st ed. Pass Test; 2006.

Raftery AT. Churchill's Pocketbook of Surgery, 2nd ed. Edinburgh: Churchill Livingstone; 2001.

Raftery AT, Delbridge MS. Basic Science for MRCS, 1st ed. Edinburgh: Churchill Livingstone; 2006.

SIGN Guideline 46: Early Management of Head Injury.

SIGN Guideline 48: Management of early rheumatoid arthritis.

SIGN Guideline 56: Prevention and management of hip fracture in older people.

SIGN Guideline 71: Management of osteoporosis.

Snaith M. ABC of Rheumatology, 3rd ed. London: BMJ Books; 2002.

Solomon L, Warwick D, Nayagam S. Apley's concise system of orthopaedics and fractures, 3rd ed. London: Hodder Arnold; 2005.

Surgery. Elsevier: Medicine Publishing. 24:11 November 2006.

Surgery. Elsevier: Medicine Publishing. 24:12 December 2006.

Surgery. Elsevier: Medicine Publishing. 25:4 April 2007.

Tofield C, Milson A, Chatu S. Hands-on guide to clinical pharmacology, 2nd ed. Oxford: Blackwell Publishing; 2005.

USEFUL WEBSITES

www.rheum.med.ed.ac.uk/los/treatment: Website of the Rheumatic Diseases Unit at the University of Edinburgh with current recommendations relating to the treatment of osteoporosis.

www.rheumatology.com: For the latest information on management.

www.eemec.med.ed.ac.uk/edrug/index.asp: The eDrug formulary for the Edinburgh MBChB curriculum.

www.sign.ac.uk: For Scottish Intercollegiate Guidelines Network (SIGN) management guidelines.

INDEX

Numbers in **bold** refer to figures or tables.